— BOOK 1 —

100

Small Steps

The First 100 Pounds
You Gotta Think Right

KEITH "TEMPLE" TROTTER

NEW YORK

Book 1
100 Small Steps
The First 100 Pounds You Gotta Think Right

Published in New York, New York, by Morgan James Publishing. Morgan James and The Entrepreneurial Publisher are trademarks of Morgan James, LLC.
www.MorganJamesPublishing.com

The Morgan James Speakers Group can bring authors to your live event. For more information or to book an event visit The Morgan James Speakers Group at www.TheMorganJamesSpeakersGroup.com.

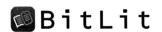

A FREE eBook edition is available
with the purchase of this print book

CLEARLY PRINT YOUR NAME IN THE BOX ABOVE

Instructions to claim your free eBook edition:
1. Download the BitLit app for Android or iOS
2. Write your name in UPPER CASE in the box
3. Use the BitLit app to submit a photo
4. Download your eBook to any device

ISBN 978-1-63047-180-4 paperback
ISBN 978-1-63047-181-1 eBook
ISBN 978-1-63047-182-8 hardcover
Library of Congress Control Number:
2014937577

Cover Design by:
Rachel Lopez
www.r2cdesign.com

Interior Design by:
Bonnie Bushman
bonnie@caboodlegraphics.com

In an effort to support local communities, raise awareness and funds, Morgan James Publishing donates a percentage of all book sales for the life of each book to Habitat for Humanity Peninsula and Greater Williamsburg.

Get involved today, visit
www.MorganJamesBuilds.com.

Habitat
for Humanity®
Peninsula and
Greater Williamsburg
Building Partner

1

'And now, to announce the award for best television lighting, it's my proud honour to present to you that much-loved zany comic actor, Dermot Donnelly!'

An implausibly vigorous burst of clapping erupted from amongst the tightly packed tables as a portly bucolic figure at the back struggled to make his way through to the microphones and raised dais. TV cameras followed his Womble-like movements.

'Who the bloody hell's Dermot Donnelly?' demanded Philip Fletcher, in a voice like frazzled thunder.

'Ssh!' hissed Seymour Loseby, who was sitting beside him. 'Keep clapping, dear! I think camera three may be about to traverse across us.'

Philip weakly flapped one palm against the other. He couldn't have shown much more enthusiasm even had he wanted to – his skin was practically chafed to the bone. It was ten o'clock, they'd been there for three hours and they hadn't even started on the major awards yet. The acting awards, naturally. Philip didn't give a damn about the rest.

Not that he was up for a prize himself this year (though everyone with any discernment knew that he should have been) but if he wasn't in line to receive anything it became doubly important that neither of the two cretins brain-bogglingly nominated for Best Actor got anything either. The incompetence of the hapless wretches assigned to the awards committee staggered him. Had anyone present

7

been kind enough to lend him a loaded machine gun, he just wouldn't have known where to start.

'Dick Jones is looking nervous,' Seymour murmured.

On the other hand . . .

Jones was sitting four tables away, conveniently next to one of the open channels used by the all-too-infrequent waiters, ready at an instant to answer the summons to immortality. A particularly gormless minor Royal was on bauble duty tonight, passing out the job lot of imitation gilt statuettes with all the aplomb of a car-park attendant dispensing tickets. Dick Jones was revving up to go.

'Wonder how long he took over his acceptance speech,' Seymour whispered in Philip's ear.

Philip laughed sourly. The public seemed to think that a quick scribble on the back of a napkin was all it took, but that was strictly for the amateurs, and whatever else you might say about Dick Jones, he was no amateur. When Philip had been nominated for the same award a few years previously he'd spent days over his speech, writing and rewriting the script endlessly in his head, practising to death all those little inflections, pauses; the candid freshness and the choked humility that are the marks of the seasoned pro. American actors tend to straddle the tightrope of emotion, quivering between tears and laughter as they display the full extent of their all-embracing human wondrousness, while the English affect a casual unconcerned air in keeping with an anachronistic view of the national character perpetuated, ironically, by images from the silver screen. But in both cases the aim is the same – to keep the tension between text and subtext sublimely balanced, to offset the gentle voice sobbing to the spotlights, 'I am not worthy,' with the screamed whisper, 'OH YES I BLOODY WELL AM!'

Unfortunately Philip had never had the chance to deliver his version. Instead the prize that year had gone to a shaggy youth with a charisma vacuum called Rufus Bohun, whose

8

entry form for Best of Breeds at Cruft's must have been dispatched to the wrong address. The error had been compounded, for Bohun was up for it again this year, along with Jones and three perfectly acceptable if uninspiring mediocrities. At all costs one of the mediocrities had to win. Philip was consoled by the thought that one usually did.

Dermot Donnelly had cracked his expected quota of completely unfunny jokes and was shaking hands with a boffin-type who'd just been over to receive his award from the dim-looking duchess. The boffin-type took a hesitant step towards the microphone, but was expertly steered away by some hovering minions, who were under strict instructions not to allow speechifying from anyone with a below-the-line credit. Had it been otherwise, the already fractious and fatigued guests would have had to book themselves in for breakfast.

'Thanks, Dermot!' said the female compere for the evening, who was showing as much cleavage to the cameras as her plastic surgeon had been able to rig up for her.

'Love that hat!' chipped in the male compere by her side.

Dermot Donnelly wasn't wearing a hat, but some of the audience laughed and the zany comic grabbed at his bald pate with an agonized expression. Philip smiled mirthlessly at the witless 'catchphrase'. He was beginning to feel like a Mensa observer at a Retards' Night Out.

'Thanks again, Dermot!' the male compere grinned. Everything he said was accompanied by a grin. His over-tanned *crème brûlée* face was so stretched with permanently dyed laugh lines it looked as if someone had just shoved a broom handle up his rear end. If they hadn't, Philip was ready to oblige.

'Yes, thanks, Dermot!' said his co-host, taking a quick squint at a card in her hand to remind herself of what came next.

9

The evening's torture would have been over ages ago, Philip reflected, if the comperes hadn't felt constrained to repeat everything at least three times. Unfortunately they had been culled from the list of daytime television presenters, at a time when cuts in broadcasters' budgets had resulted in a strict ration of one shared brain cell per pair. Needless to say, their egos were in inverse proportion to their IQs.

'And now, before we get to hear the nominations for Best Supporting Actors,' the pneumatic hostess was saying, having finished mugging from her card, 'we have a very special treat lined up. Ladies and gentlemen, will you please put your hands together, give a big round of applause and a very special showbiz welcome to that ever-popular singing star who's flown in especially to be with us here tonight, Mr Ricky Rix with his special guests the Garry Goetz Dancers!'

The tired and dispirited audience put their raw bleeding palms together unenthusiastically. Philip imagined the TV director in the editing suite frantically amplifying the applause. If only he could find a way of drowning out the noise of Ricky Rix at the same time (whoever he was) he would deserve the thanks of a grateful nation.

The general lighting dimmed and prerecorded music began to seep from some giant speakers. The stage at the back of the banqueting hall started to tremble as the dance troupe took up their positions with slick hippopotamic grace. Suddenly a single white spot began twitching across the floor, and, as the orchestral intro burst into a luscious climax, a rotund gnome in a silver suit bounced into view and started whining into a microphone. A beat late on cue, coloured lights flashed across the back of the stage and the line of dancers commenced cavorting. Philip discreetly put his hands over his ears.

Unfortunately he didn't have any spare appendages to put over his eyes at the same time. The assault on his remaining unblinkered senses continued apace, lightened only by an exchange of theatrical winces with his fellow table guests. The tubby second-rater up on stage continued his off-key warble, supported by an out-of-step flabby-thighed line of overage kickers who looked as if they'd be hard put to come fourth in a regional qualifying heat of *Come Dancing*. It was excruciating and, much worse, it was plain embarrassing. When it came to Awards ceremonies the British just didn't have a clue. The menu had been copied from a transatlantic original, but with tinned ingredients substituted for fresh produce. The style and the dash had evaporated, only the vulgarity remained. All that glistered was fool's gold.

The food, naturally, had been cold on arrival, and the miserable ration of *vinaigre de table* long since consumed. Philip wondered if the evening had been sponsored by the Temperance League. At least he had had the foresight to bring his own hip flask. Next time he came to one of these bashes he would have to remember to fill it with hemlock.

At long last the sad but criminally overpaid crooner finished his painful wail, the chorus line took their last uncoordinated toe-poke at the air, and a silence punctuated only by the fitful scratchings and stirrings of two hundred desperately bored people was resumed. Someone gave the male compere a nudge and his face lit and froze like a tilted pinball table. He began gushing automatically into the nearest TV camera.

'Thanks, Ricky, that was terrific! And now, ladies and gentlemen, we move ever nearer to the climax of tonight's proceedings. To announce the nominations for Best Supporting Actress, will you please give a great big hand to . . .'

A kind of white noise had infiltrated Philip's brain. He had been asked to give too many big hands already, he had heard announced the names of too many alleged celebrities whose prior existence he had never remotely guessed at. He was so utterly bored that he felt almost transcendent;

11

he was sure that any moment now he would begin floating to the ceiling. He could no longer even go through the motions of appreciation. Time, which had seemed merely to be going like a snail, now went like a crab, backwards. Another breath of this oxygen-starved air and his whole life would begin to flash before him.

An unknown man came to the microphone and spoke. There was more clapping, there were gasps, there were cheers, and a middle-aged actress gushed on to the stage to clutch tearfully at the proffered statuette. A pause, another fatuous exchange between the comperes, and another actress was introduced to go through the same procedures, a rite worn smooth and leading by inexorable degree to the familiar lifeless clap, the notional gasp, the hollow cheer and the plastic grin on the recipient's face. The new-crowned Best Supporting Actor gave the air a punch and came back down from the Olympian heights. The next envelope was readied and the next thespian summoned from the taxi ranks below to open it. Seymour Loseby gave Philip a nudge. He dimly registered the words coming from the podium.

'. . . Natasha Fielding, for her performance as Cleopatra in *Antony and Cleopatra* . . .'

The time capsule had ceased its counter-clockwise motion. Fragments of memory reassembled in Philip's consciousness. Natasha's face filled his mind's eye, her voice his inner ear. He almost quivered at her imagined touch. For the first time in many a long hour his smile was unforced.

'I can't make it, darling,' she had murmured coyly on the phone, long-distance from her chosen outpost of exile in the Canadian wilderness. 'I mean, it's starting to show. You'll have to go for me.'

In the infertile northern fastness her belly at least was ripening. She had decided that her child should be born in the Arctic twilight, as far away as possible from the public eye. And an equivalent distance, too, from the natural father, who nonetheless still found himself dragooned into acting as her substitute. His presence there tonight, Philip reflected, showed a devotion way beyond the call of duty. And in return for what, pray? he asked himself wryly. What was his reward for having allowed himself to be so comprehensively twisted round Natasha Fielding's littlest finger? What was in it for him?

The chance to bask in reflected glory? Ha! Natasha's nomination for Best Actress might or might not be deserved (he supposed that it was) but where was his own corresponding accolade? Despite the critics' inexcusable indifference he knew that his Antony had been a first-rate performance and, moreover, that it had been he who had carried the initially lacklustre Natasha. She'd only begun to spark into life the night she'd murdered her lover, which he supposed he ought to have taken as a warning shot across the bows in the light of their subsequent relationship. But events had passed much too quickly, much too dramatically, to allow him time for considered reflection. His only thought had been to cover up the murder and conceal the body, a process in which, despite his wide expertise in nefarious activities, he had come perilously close to discovery. And what had been the result? Not a victory in his long-running theatrical feud with Dick Jones, that was for sure. There was Jones now, waiting to see if his miserable name was the one stencilled inside the unopened envelope. Thankfully he was up for some modern studio play he'd done at the beginning of last year, and not for the National's own appalling production of *Antony and Cleopatra*, for which, to Philip's eternal humiliation and disgust, Jones had been selected ahead of him. But it was a small mercy. In the great scheme of things Jones's star was in the ascendant, while Philip was cast as lackey, stand-in, spear carrier, and, worst of all, prospective parent. The other roles he might be able to swallow, but not that one. It was still a moot point with him which had been Natasha's meanest trick, the mere fact of her using him as a sperm bank for uncredited withdrawals, or the ensuing fiction that the actual progenitor had been her murdered lover, the late and by no means lamented Sergei Shustikov. Not that Philip possessed even the merest glimmer of a paternal instinct, but, nonetheless, he did possess the instinct of an artist, and he regarded correct billing as a sacrosanct contractual obligation. Damn it all, he may not have been consulted over the issue, but it was his handiwork. It went against the grain to allow another to take the bow.

'And the winner is . . . Natasha Fielding, for Cleopatra!'

Seymour's roar in his ear jolted him away from his thoughts. He heard the man on stage speak his name.

'Sadly, Natasha can't be with us tonight. So will you please give a warm welcome to Philip Fletcher, who's here to accept the award on her behalf.'

Philip rose stiffly. The applause, which in other circumstances he would have found gratifying, was irksome. It was not for him.

'So *that's* why I'm here!' he murmured sourly to Seymour as he left the table. 'I had wondered . . .'

Serenely, Philip wound his way up to the raised dais, to the accompaniment of his peers' applause and the powerful strings of echt-Mantovani swelling from the on-stage speakers. He sprang on to the platform, bobbed his head at the duchess as he scooped the statuette up in his arms, pretended to hear the pearl of dross she dropped from her lips, and then turned smartly to the real focus of his attention, the microphone. He nestled in behind it and tilted his chin upwards, for the benefit of the cameras. The applause died away.

'Thank you so very, very much,' he said, with aching surrogate sincerity. 'It's a terrible tragedy Natasha can't be here with all her friends tonight . . .'

He paused, for well-judged effect. He'd just spotted one of Natasha's 'friends' in the front row, Lindsay Leonard, another of the shortlisted actresses and yet another of his distinguished ex-co-stars. The flash of undiluted loathing in her eye was wondrous to behold. He felt a mischievous urge to divulge the real reason for Natasha's absence. Oh, did he have a tale to tell to the yet unknowing world! Talk of accidental murders and casual slaughters . . .

'I know that Natasha will feel honoured, privileged, utterly thrilled, and yet, somehow at the same time, completely humbled to receive this wonderful award . . .'

Philip glanced down at the naff statuette. He hoped the cheap gilt paint wasn't about to start coming off on his palms.

'Much, indeed, as I felt when I first learnt I was to star opposite this marvellous, extraordinarily talented and, dare I say, breathtakingly beautiful actress . . .'

He paused to enjoy the sight of Lindsay Leonard's face turning livid purple. He wondered just how much more of this crap she'd be able to take before steam started coming out of her ears. He decided it might be fun to find out.

'Her vivid and inspirational performance is as fresh and vibrant in my imagination tonight as it was on that first electric evening in Hammersmith more than six months ago. Hammersmith, Hammersmith . . . it may lack the ring of Stratford, the glamour of Shaftesbury Avenue, the style of Broadway, the panache of the *Comédie Française*, the reputation of the *Berliner Ensemble*, the pedigree of the Moscow Arts Theatre, yet I truly and profoundly believe deep within my heart of hearts, that for the duration of our run that humble postal district of West London was quite transformed. It is a truly rare thing for an actor to step on to the stage and feel that he is in the presence of greatness, that a page in that rare and priceless book of theatrical history is about to be turned, that another name is set to be writ up there in flaming neon alongside Terry,

Bernhardt, Duse, but yet – and I say this without the slightest fear of exaggeration – I had not the least doubt that I was in the presence of another addition to that august and noble pantheon of immortal thespian heroines. Nor do I believe that any of my peers shared for a moment the least doubt either.'

'Hear! hear!' called out Seymour from the pit.

Philip gave a restrained smile. Lindsay Leonard's grip on the edge of her tablecloth was so hard that he wondered if they'd ever be able to prise her fingers away from it. Her eyes were aglow with daggers of the mind.

'As you know, very sadly Natasha can't be with us here tonight, but it would be invidious to pass over the occasion without giving praise where praise is due, and thanking all those wonderful people without whose support Natasha's, and indeed my own (humble) performance, and our whole joyous but essentially tragic sojourn in "Hammersmith", could not have taken place. It's a long list, but I make no apologies. Short cuts are anathema to the artist, and I know that you will bear with me while I acknowledge all those to whom acknowledgement is not merely merited but also necessary . . .'

When Philip at length descended, a long five minutes later, he experienced a powerful sense of what it must have been like in the wake of a three-day bombardment on the Somme: the shell-shocked glaze in everyone's eyes, the hopelessness implicit in the slumped shoulders and sagging chins, the almost tangible miasma of despair floating about the room – he wouldn't have been at all surprised to see white napkins being waved in surrender above the tables. It had been a merciless and remorseless barrage.

'That should have softened 'em up for Dick Jones,' Philip murmured maliciously to Seymour as he resumed his place.

Way before the end of his interminable speech Philip had noticed the evening's organizers in anxious conference.

16

Whoever it was who won Best Actor, he was bound to be cut short. A minor triumph, certainly, but the best that Philip could hope to engineer in the circumstances.

'And now, to announce the final award, for Best Actor, will you please give a warm welcome to last year's Best Actress, the ever-popular and evergreen Diana Lewis!'

'Evergreen?' Seymour muttered incredulously into Philip's ear over the applause. 'Eversloshed, more like, the raddled old bat!'

'She speaks very highly of you, too, Seymour,' replied Philip, who was thinking that an underweight gnat would be hard put to get sloshed on tonight's alcoholic allowance. Diana Lewis did a little curtsey to the duchess and picked up the white envelope from the comperes. Philip held his breath as she pulled out the card.

'The nominations for Best Actor are: Rufus Bohun for *Coriolanus* at the Donmar Warehouse; David Ewart for Newton in *Sacred Geometry* at the Pit; Richard Jones for Ken in *Incontinence* at the Royal Court . . .'

Philip sat perfectly still. The white noise had returned, an aural fog which buzzed around his head. Diana Lewis was taking an age to read the other names.

'And the winner is . . .'

Jones was staring intently at the tablecloth, giving a rather poor impression of a man unconcerned. Philip was staring at Jones.

'. . . David Ewart for Newton!'

'Yes!' Philip screamed ecstatically, driving his tender palms into each other with manic abandon. 'Oh yes!'

He could hardly contain himself. He wanted to leap on to the table and perform a victory jig; he wanted to seize hold of David Ewart on his way up to the dais and smother him with kisses. Had he been struck down at that moment he would have died a happy man.

'Steady on,' Seymour murmured at him. 'Jones'll hear you.'

17

'Bugger Jones!'

It looked as though someone already had. He was sitting at his table, weakly but unconvincingly joining in the applause for David Ewart, the thinnest smile imaginable pulling at the corners of his mouth. A look of utter sour disgust was erupting through his pores.

'Hallelujah!' Philip cried, sinking back into his seat in a state of bliss. 'Good old Ewart! Bloody wonderful!'

He reached instinctively for his glass, but there was nothing in it.

'A pity,' Seymour nodded. 'I feel that Ewart deserves a toast.'

'Too right. Well, this'll all be over in a minute, thank God! I hope it's not too late to go somewhere.'

'I know a place. Might not be your cup of tea, though, Philip.'

Philip laughed sardonically.

'My dear old thing, a cup of tea is the last thing on my mind. It's champagne on me tonight!'

2

'To success!' said Seymour, tilting his glass of champagne.
'And failure,' added Philip with relish. 'Though not our
own!'

He was in a thoroughly jolly mood tonight. The ludicrously expensive warm fake champagne could not
impugn it; nor even the ludicrously warm fake-expensive
surroundings.

He had known, of course, precisely what Seymour's
warnings would entail. 'Not quite your cup of tea' was a
euphemism to conjure with. A cup of crème de menthe
might have been more descriptive.

Philip, despite a working lifetime spent in the backstage
demi-monde, had never before encountered so much concentrated campery. The smoky entrance hall, decorated
only with a monochrome portrait of Lord Alfred Douglas
(the lips, though, touched up with screaming vermilion),
had given away little, but the steps going down to the
basement under the curly neon club name, Bosie Butterflys, had led them into an exotic fairy grotto. Every surface
was gilded and curved; every face was encrusted with
powder and rouge. And that was just the waiters. The
alcoves which circled the room (and in one of which they
sat) were marked off by alabaster Doric pillars and fes-
tooned with acres of crimson velvet drape. More velvet
hung from the ceilings, gathered and bunched then drip-
ping in cascades of rich material down almost to head

height. The small stage at the back, opposite the silver and black horseshoe bar, was shaped and painted like a seashell, and finished in translucent salmon, though the elaborate lighting bathed everything in a Hammerish, blood-red glow.

'Is that just for show?' Philip had enquired, nodding towards the stage.

'Oh no, there's a cabaret!'

Philip couldn't wait. More to the point, nor could Seymour.

'We're in for a very special treat tonight!' he confided to Philip eagerly. 'Doris is performing herself.'

'Doris?'

'Doris Afternoon. Doris is the manager.'

Philip had nothing to say. The name said it all really.

'Anything on the work front?' Seymour asked, sipping champagne.

'Mm? Oh, um, not a lot . . .'

Philip was momentarily distracted by the sight of a distinguished-looking elderly man in a conservative suit tweaking the leather posing pouch of one of the waiters. The elderly man was a well-known theatrical impresario.

'No, nothing on the horizon, but frankly I'm glad of a break.'

'Filming took it out of you?'

'Yes.'

He had gone almost straight from the stage run of *Antony and Cleopatra* into a hectic six-week shooting schedule, playing a sex-starved country parson in a steamy TV adaptation of a bestselling aga saga. Now that Natasha had exited so suddenly from his life, the sex-starved bit hadn't required a lot of acting. And things weren't going to get any better on that front if he spent too much more of his spare time hanging round Bosie Butterflys.

'Do you come here often?' he asked facetiously.

'Yes. I should warn you – it's full of poufs.'

20

'You don't say.'

'My reputation must be in tatters. Cooee! Sandy!' The object of his attentions, a thin gingery waiter who was carrying a tray of drinks, paused, pirouetted, and waved gaily back before continuing on his way.

'Such a nice boy,' Seymour murmured, discreetly holding out his forefingers in front of him, six inches or so apart. '*That* big . . .'

'I think it's my reputation we have to worry about, Seymour. Yours is long gone.'

'I should care, at my age?'

'You'll outlive us all.'

'Then I shall look forward to delivering your funeral oration. What should you like me to say?'

'As I shan't be there, I really couldn't care.'

'No eye for posterity, Philip?'

'I'm not sure I care for the morbid turn this conversation has taken.'

'But what if they renamed a theatre after you? Surely you'd be flattered!'

'How can a corpse be flattered?'

'You're being very literal-minded tonight. I bet Dick Jones would jump at the idea.'

'Now you've descended from the morbid to the banal. I shall have to rinse away the foul taste in my mouth with another draught of champagne. You on for another bottle?'

Seymour hesitated. He patted his heart gently.

'The quack says to go easy on the booze. Really I shouldn't.'

'I'll get a half-bottle then.'

'I only said I shouldn't, Philip. That doesn't mean I won't. Make it a big one. I may have that phrase inscribed on my tombstone.'

'Oh, for heaven's sake! I feel like I'm in an Ingmar Bergman film; it's like having a drink with Death. Any moment now you'll get your chess set out.'

'Black bishop takes white queen. Mm, there's an idea.'

'I'm glad to see your thoughts directed back into the earthly sphere. Thanks, Sandy.'

The waiter left the bottle standing in the ice bucket and departed. Philip tasted the champagne suspiciously.

'I think it's lemonade.'

'At least it'll wash the foul taste from your mouth.'

'I'm sorry?'

'The taste of Dick Jones.'

'You will keep lowering the tone, Seymour. Still, the picture on his face was priceless.'

'You might not be so pleased in the New Year, Philip.'

'We've only just started a new year. What do you mean?'

'I'm talking about the next one. The Honours List. Rumour has it that Jones is in line for a gong; he only just missed out this time.'

'Well, you can tell the country's going to the dogs. They'll give an MBE to anyone these days.'

'It's a lot worse than that, Philip. I understand he may be up for a big one.'

'A big one? What do you . . . ? You don't mean – you can't mean!'

'I'm afraid I can. Tap on the shoulder time.'

'What?'

'Sir Richard Jones. Not got much of a ring, has it?'

'WHAT?'

'Philip, are you all right? You're looking very pale.'

It was hardly surprising; he could actually feel the blood evacuating his cheeks. It was still pounding through his brain, though, he could feel that too: a pummelling through the temples, an explosive thump-thump in his ears. The noise was overwhelming, he felt disoriented. Then he realized that he was hearing music, loud and tinny. He became aware of something nudging him in the ribs. It was Seymour's elbow.

'It's show time!' announced his friend. 'Sit back and enjoy!'

The lights dimmed and the rhythm beating into Philip's head intensified. The music, a lushly swelling show tune, was coming from the speakers either side of the stage. A man in a dinner jacket bounded up on to the translucent pink seashell and seized the microphone.

'Ladies and gentlemen, will you give a very, very warm Bosie Butterflys welcome to our very own queen of the cabaret, the mega-talented and ever-delectable Miss Doris Afternoon!'

A powerful wave of applause flooded up to the stage. A pair of bright white profile spots shone through the bloody glow to illuminate the microphone. The drapes at the back parted and a man in a dress tottered out on high heels.

The man in the dress was already six foot plus in his fishnetted feet; in heels he was a true Goliath among female impersonators. The curls of his peroxide beehive wig brushed almost against the ceiling, but his excess of scale was by no means confined to the vertical plane – great wads of fat bulged out on all sides. When he inclined his head to acknowledge his adoring public his chins multiplied exponentially. A fist like a pork butcher's seized hold of the microphone.

'What a lovely welcome!' he growled in a throaty parody of vampishness. He fluttered his inch-long lashes: 'And what a lovely lot you are!'

There was a further bout of satisfied cheering. Someone gave an ineffective wolf-whistle. The wolf in sheep's clothing up on stage batted a few eyelashes.

'Blow dear, don't suck.'

As the roar of knowing laughter subsided a camera flash went off. Doris Afternoon looked archly in the direction of the photographer.

'Come back and see me afterwards; I'll show you how to do an enlargement.'

As the hoots and catcalls faded a thin bald man in tails entered and sat himself down at an upright piano by the side of the stage.

'I would say give Norman a big hand, but knowing him he wouldn't give it back afterwards. Let's have a tinkle, maestro!'

Norman smiled sourly. He gave the ivories a flourish. Doris Afternoon gave a dismissive wave.

'Enough of this banter. No more tittle-tattle.'

He thrust his spare hand under his bra and gave his massive padded bosoms an upward thrust.

'More tittle, less tattle, eh? That's what Norman always says. Eh, dear?'

Norman banged out some flowery chords. Somewhere along the line they must have turned into an intro, because Doris Afternoon launched suddenly into 'Somewhere Over the Rainbow'.

Judy Garland it wasn't.

The audience loved it, though. Barely had the screams of 'Encore!' and 'Bravo!' died down than Doris had begun the next number. 'Hey, Big Spender!' was followed by Noel Coward's 'Nina', and then, with an even more startling absence of continuity, by 'I've Got a Lovely Bunch of Coconuts'. The audience was encouraged to join in the refrain.

'I'll bet you have!' Doris would say each time, holding out the microphone to pick up a likely-looking communal warbler. Seymour's contribution, delivered with what one could only term gay abandon, attracted a nod from onstage.

'We all know about you, dear!' muttered Doris Afternoon, giving him an arch wink. Seymour gave every appearance of wanting to roll over on his back and wave his legs in the air.

'That's enough of that, Norman!' said Doris curtly, as the pianist lingered over a final rococo twirl. The singer bathed in the applause unaccompanied.

'You've been a lovely audience!' he cooed. He simpered as he caught the eye of a brawny leather-clad man who was returning to his seat: 'Some more lovely than others . . . I'll catch you later!'

Doris Afternoon backed off delicately through the curtains, blowing kisses at the ecstatic audience. Someone threw a loose bouquet of tulips on to the stage. Doris affected a blush and exited in an unlikely display of modesty.

'Isn't she wonderful!' Seymour yelled in Philip's ear over the thunderous clapping.

'Highly original,' Philip answered distractedly. His mind had been largely engaged elsewhere during the performance.

'Sandy! Sandy, love!'

The waiter noticed Seymour's frantic waving and made his way over.

'Sandy, tell Doris I'd love to buy her a drink. She knows I'm here.'

'I'll bet she does,' answered Sandy knowingly. 'Everyone knows you're here!'

The waiter promised to pass on the message. Seymour took the opportunity to order another bottle.

'I thought you had to go easy?' queried Philip.

'Don't be a spoilsport. I'm having much too good a time. Why aren't you?'

'Sorry?'

'For heaven's sake, Philip, why are you looking so glum? Anyone would think Dick Jones had actually won Best Actor!'

'He might just as well have done.'

'What?'

'Where'd you hear this about the Honours List?'

'From the boy. But don't tell a soul I told you. It's confidential.'

'You're sure about it?'

'I'm only going on what I've been told, dear. But the boy's track record is pretty good in these matters.'

Unfortunately, Philip couldn't doubt it. The 'boy' was Nigel Loseby, Seymour's son. It was startling enough that Seymour should have ever sired an offspring ('a bit of a cock-up' was his own description of the aberrant coupling), but what was doubly astonishing was that the boy, now thirtysomething pushing forty, should have turned out to be such a rigorously upstanding and outstanding pillar of the community: a Conservative MP for ten years now and darling of the Right, once the baby of the House, but already risen to junior ministerial rank and hotly tipped for the highest office in the land. Tipped by his own father, anyway, whose pride in his lad's achievements, Philip suspected, was probably not fully reciprocated.

'But . . .' Philip waved a hand uselessly. 'What in heaven's name has Jones ever done to deserve it? I mean, I know I'm biased, but there are thousands of better actors out there. What is going on?'

'I hear the PM's a fan. He had to take some foreign dignitaries to the RSC a few years ago, and Jones was the star turn. I gather he made a big impression at the reception afterwards.'

'It must have been more convincing than his impression of a classical actor.'

'Too true, I fear. The boy is of the opinion that the PM knows rather more about the delivery of off-spin bowling than Shakespearian verse. Apparently Jones has done some flag-flying abroad. There's a lot of gong-grade mileage in British Council tours.'

'Huh! Talk about patriotism as the last refuge of the scoundrel . . . I can hardly bear even to talk about this, Seymour. Sir Richard Jones! It's beyond belief. We've got to put a stop to it.'

'And how do you propose to do that? The PM's dead keen.'

'We'll have to bring down the government.'

'We *are* ambitious tonight!'

'All right, we'll lure him down here then. Get some half-naked catamite friend of yours to jump on him, take some photos and flog 'em to the *News of the World*.'

'I very much doubt if the management would approve.'

'Sod the management –'

'I wouldn't say that in such a loud voice. They're here. Doris! My darling, how lovely to see you!'

'Seymour, sweetie!' Doris Afternoon fluttered, extending a bejewelled hand in the manner of a complaisant duchess. 'My favourite thespian!'

Seymour took the proffered fist and planted a kiss on a meaty knuckle.

'May I introduce Philip Fletcher, Doris?'

'You certainly may!' answered the drag queen approvingly.

Philip felt a little self-conscious as Doris stepped back to appraise him with a shrewd eye. Should he maintain the feminine fiction? In the absence of established guidelines he supposed so; it seemed to be the done thing. He half rose as Doris waved a set of brightly painted nails under his nose.

'Charmed, Miss Afternoon,' he said politely, eschewing a kiss in favour of a simple shake of the hand. Doris gave Seymour a playful push.

'Budge up then, love. I'll never get my fat arse in there.'

Seymour moved along the padded seat and Doris Afternoon squeezed in beside him. Sandy appeared with a clean glass.

'Better get another,' commanded Doris. 'Norman is hovering with menace and looking thirsty. Chin-chin!'

Seymour clinked glasses with Doris.

'Bottoms up!'

'I'll say!'

They knocked back their champagne. Philip offered refills.

'Seems like a nice boy!' murmured Doris, giving Seymour a nudge. 'Where do you find them?'

'Where we find him is more to the point,' riposted Philip, straining a smile. Seymour sighed.

'Fletcher's irredeemably straight, I'm afraid,' he explained to Doris, then sighed again. 'You don't know what you're missing!'

Philip took a quick glance at his surroundings.

'Oh, I think I probably do . . .'

'No such thing as irredeemably straight, love,' muttered Doris, taking out a cigarette from a packet of Camel. 'Look at you!'

'At me?' said Seymour incredulously. 'I'm bent as a corkscrew!'

'That's what I mean. Every time I switch on the box there's your boy, the Honourable Member (so the rumour goes!) strutting his stuff and doing you proud! Frankly, my dear, if *you* can swing both ways, anybody can. Your friend should try it some day . . .'

'I'll bear it in mind,' Philip replied evenly. Seymour laughed.

'Can't imagine Philip here going for little boys. I'm afraid you're wasting your time.'

'Who said anything about little boys?' drawled Doris archly. 'You meet a better class of lady, Philip, in Bosie Butterflys . . .'

The drag queen leant low across the table towards him, pushing a well-stuffed bosom along the shiny surface. A leer spread across the brightly daubed face, cracking the powdered skin and revealing the crow-lines beneath. A row of gold-capped teeth glittered in the half-light. The glint in the eyes had the same hard metallic lustre.

Not the most appetizing offer he'd ever had, Philip

reflected. He settled back in his seat languidly and took out a cigarette of his own.

'I think I'll stick to what I know,' he said, discreetly thumbing the wheel on his lighter to maximum then producing a sudden violent spurt of flame in the space between them. Doris sat back sharply.

'Terribly sorry,' murmured Philip, toning it down and lighting his own cigarette.

'You should be careful with that thing,' said Doris, a shade crossly. 'It's not bonfire night, you know.'

'Then why all the Halloween masks?' Philip looked at his watch. 'It's late, I think I'll make tracks.'

It was late, but he wasn't tired and the hour was irrelevant. He was finding the atmosphere in the club claustrophobic, and the presence of the tarted-up old sham sitting opposite frankly nauseous. A strict immoralist himself, in the normal run of things he couldn't care less what other people got up to, what they did, with whom, when, where, why. He was as fond of Seymour Loseby as of anybody, he had no axe to grind, no judgement to weigh, neither approval nor disapproval to voice in any wise. If anyone should and did exist by a philosophy of Live and Let Live it was he. But something about Doris Afternoon got on his nerves. Not so much the over-made-up vulgarity, nor even the remorseless drip of double entendres (though he did feel like he was in the remake of *Carry On Camping*), but, specifically, it was an acute sense of the character beneath the pancake and powder that deterred him. Doris Afternoon, or whatever the hell he was called really, came over as a calculating mean-eyed little shit.

'Good night, Seymour,' said Philip, feigning a yawn and extracting some notes from his wallet. 'It's been a lovely evening.'

'Let me contribute,' said his friend, reaching for an inside pocket, but Philip raised a hand sharply:

'No, no, drinks on me – I did say!'

29

He dropped four fifty-pound notes on to the table. At over sixty pounds a bottle, it would barely cover the bill. And he was leaving a full glass of the lemonade substitute undrunk. He felt like he'd just been mugged.

'Lovely to meet you,' said Doris Afternoon, extending a hand. Reluctantly Philip took it, and felt his fingers being tickled. 'Come again – as I say to all my satisfied customers!'

Philip couldn't even be bothered to pretend to smile. He squeezed himself out from under the table.

'Is Sandy around?' Seymour asked. 'If you see him on your way out, could you say we need some more drinks?'

'What was all this guff about having to go easy?' Philip demanded. 'At this rate you'll drink the place dry.'

'Seymour always likes to suck things dry,' drawled Doris Afternoon.

'You're a fine one to talk!' exclaimed Seymour. 'Oh, Philip!'

Philip had started to go. He stopped and turned back expectantly. Seymour rummaged deep in his black leather shoulder-bag, which he had deposited on the floor beside him. 'Aren't you forgetting something?'

Seymour opened the bag and spilled the contents across the table: pills, keys, tissues, a thick book with hard plain red covers and, last of all, the small imitation gilt statuette – Natasha's prize – entrusted to him earlier for safe keeping. Doris Afternoon was unable to resist fingering the hermaphroditic figurine.

'No one I know . . . Don't want to take anything away from you, Philip, but I was always told it was bad manners to come first.'

Philip ignored him.

'Thanks, Seymour. I'll be in touch.'

Seymour was putting his things back into the shoulder-bag. Doris picked up the thick red book.

'My, you must know a lot of people! Biggest I've ever seen!'

'I bet you say that to all the boys,' Seymour answered.

'I mean the address book, silly!'

'What else could you mean?'

'Don't make me blush!'

'As if I could!'

Seymour gave the red book a pat before returning it to his bag. He winked at them both.

'There's more than just addresses in here, you know. An intimate journal of record. You'd be shocked and surprised.'

'I'm unshockable.'

'I know you are. Philip might not be, though.'

'I'm not sure I can believe *that*,' said Doris suggestively, attempting to catch Philip's eye and inveigle him back into a further round of raillery. But Philip wasn't prepared to bite.

'Speak to you soon, Seymour,' he said over his shoulder, hurrying off. It seemed to have taken forever to make his farewells, and he'd just caught a glimpse of Norman, the pianist, making his way through the throng to join them. It was imperative he make his exit before he was dragged into another round of introductions.

He stopped only to relay Seymour's drinks order to Sandy and to reclaim his coat from the cloakroom. The club was located in a side street off Tottenham Court Road; it took him a frustrating few minutes to find signs of cosmopolitan life and a taxi. He sat in the back solemnly on the way to Highbury, nursing the little gilt statuette, and his grievances.

He ignored the junk mail in the hall and took the stairs directly to his first-floor flat. He unfastened the double-locked doors and made his way quickly to the wall cabinet to switch off the alarm. It was already off. He'd been late leaving, he supposed that he must have been in too much of a hurry to set it. He gave the room a quick check, though,

31

to be on the safe side. Nothing appeared to have been disturbed.

He threw off his coat, flung open the bedroom door and switched on the light. He stopped suddenly, in the middle of loosening his bow tie.

Someone was sleeping in his bed.

3

The shape in the bed moved. Philip nervously brandished the gilt statuette.

'Don't move – I'm armed!'

The duvet was flung back, and a thin black body clad only in a pair of red boxer shorts leapt out and staggered to attention beside the bed. The two huge globular eyes which blinked back at him looked as if they were about to burst with panic.

'You what?'

'I don't . . . George!'

Philip's arm fell limply to his side, in sympathy with his dropping jaw. He didn't know whether to erupt in fury or laughter.

'George, would you mind telling me what you are doing here, please?' he asked, with what he considered to be, in the circumstances, commendable restraint.

'Er . . .'

George didn't quite seem all there yet. While he stood scratching his head, Philip wandered over to the dresser and put down the statuette.

'You're very lucky, George,' he remarked coolly. 'I might have brained you, like last time.'

It had been over a year ago that Philip had interrupted the young delinquent in the act of burgling his flat. The youth's attempted flight (impeded by the weight of the just-stolen video recorder) had been arrested emphatically

33

by Philip smashing a whisky bottle over his head. It had been an inauspicious start to a relationship which, surprisingly, had blossomed to their mutual advantage.

'I thought you were meant to be in Manchester?' Philip offered, hoping to kickstart the boy's fuzzy mental processes back into life.

'Got a week off,' George answered. He broke for a full-blooded yawn before adding: 'Half term.'

After a brief course of one-on-one lessons Philip had engineered George's entry into drama school. He was actually midway through the first year of a degree course, which, considering the shortcomings in both his talent and education, was no mean feat. Philip was impressed that he'd stuck it out.

'I see. So you came straight back to London?'

'Yeah.'

'Whereupon, naturally enough, you immediately broke into my flat?'

'I didn't break nothing! I came through the window. Look! It ain't broke, is it?'

Philip opened the window and peered outside. The ledge was narrow, and the drainpipe, up which he had shimmied, barely secure.

'I should know by now that it's your preferred mode of entry. I suppose I should congratulate you on your athleticism and dexterity.'

''Ere! Close that, can't you? It's bloody freezing!'

Philip obligingly reclosed the window and cast a semi-amused glance at the shivering naked figure by the bed.

'Awfully sorry to discomfit you ... What did you do about the alarm?'

'I know where you keep the key. Under the ashtray.'

'Yes, I thought it was on. Well, I'm glad you didn't have to disable it, anyway. As I know full well you can.'

'Yeah ...' George laughed. He picked a sweatshirt out

of a pile of clothes on the floor and put it on. 'That was a hairy one, eh?'

Philip nodded. The night they'd burgled Ken Kilmaine's office had been one of the hairiest of his career. He couldn't have done it without George. Still, that didn't mean he had to welcome him with open arms at the present moment.

'Why didn't you go to your uncle's?'

George's uncle and aunt were his legal guardians, his mother long ago having conceded that her parental responsibilities were impossible to discharge. They lived the other side of Highbury Grove.

'They ain't in. I dunno where they got to.'

'Don't you have a key?'

'I lost it.'

'So you resorted instinctively to housebreaking. What's wrong with their place? What were you doing in my bed?'

'Sleeping. Till you came in.'

'I apologize for my lack of consideration.'

George had picked his watch off the bedside table. He was examining it incredulously.

'It's two o'clock! Where you been?'

'If you must know, I've been to a gay night club.'

'You what?'

George stared at him suspiciously.

'I didn't think you was like that . . .'

'No, it's a new thing with me. If you'd like to get back into bed now, I'll be with you shortly.'

The expression on George's face finally made Philip's night worthwhile. George stared at him sulkily while he abandoned himself to uproarious laughter.

'Ain't that funny,' he muttered at length, when Philip had strained his diaphragm to the limit. 'How's I supposed to know you wasn't coming back?'

'Just because I'm not using my bed, that doesn't mean I'm happy to let you use it.'

'What was I supposed to do? Sleep on the floor?'

35

'Well, that's precisely what you're going to have to do now. Use the sofa, it's perfectly comfortable, I've slept there myself. There are some blankets in the cupboard. Help yourself. I've got to make a phone call.'

'A phone call? Who you ringing at this time of night?'

'None of your business.'

Philip went back into the living room, feeling on the whole slightly more amused than irritated. George's impertinence aside, he felt perversely pleased to see him. Despondency was weighing heavily on him tonight. He was glad of some company.

The number he wanted was on a letter he had left lying by the phone. He consulted his telephone book for the correct international code, settled himself back on the sofa and dialled. The letter had warned him to expect a long wait.

Eventually an elderly man answered in a thin slow voice.

'I'd like to leave a message for Natasha Fielding,' said Philip carefully. 'Is that all right?'

'She ain't here,' said the man. 'She's next door.'

'I know that,' Philip answered patiently, for the letter had explained that she would be staying in a phoneless outbuilding. 'Next door', in the context, apparently encompassed anything within a five-mile radius. 'I should like to leave a message. Have you got a pen?'

The old man at the other end gave a demented wheeze.

'What would I need a pen for, sonny? I can't read nor write!'

The old man was clearly very amused by Philip's unintended witticism; at any rate, it took him a good half-minute to stop cackling. At least it gave Philip time to master his surprise. He could appreciate that Natasha's description of her hideaway as being in 'the middle of nowhere' was no exaggeration.

'Well, can you give her a verbal message then? Could

you say Philip rang, and she won the award. You've got that? She's won the Best Actress Award.'

'Yup, she knows that.'

'Oh. Really?'

'Yup, you're the third person to ring tonight and tell me. I ain't likely to forget!'

'I see.'

Philip curled his lip. Clearly Natasha's hideaway was less brilliantly concealed than he had been led to believe. Her casual protestations of indifference to the possibility of becoming an award-winner left a *soupçon* of a credibility gap.

'Please give her my love anyway,' said Philip, over a sustained new bout of what sounded like near-terminal wheezing. He wondered if the old man would live long enough to pass on his message.

Philip put down the phone as George came in, weighed under with blankets and a sleeping bag.

'Want a coffee?' he asked his guest.

'Yeah. Cheers.'

'You'd better go and make yourself one then. I'm having a Scotch.'

Philip poured a large whisky and lit a cigarette. George stood in the kitchen doorway watching him, waiting for the kettle to boil.

'Thought you wanted to give up,' he chipped in.

'Only when there's an r in the month,' Philip answered, drawing in another lungful of carcinogens. 'I fear I'm a hopeless case. Did you manage it yourself in the end?'

George had written to him a few weeks back. The letter had been brief and contained little in the way of idle chat besides a vague line or two on the merits of a tobacco-free existence. The meat of the communication had been a rather less vague request for money. Philip had not responded.

'Ain't smoked for a month,' said George proudly. 'Voice teacher says it's bad for me.'

'I'm a bad influence, I know. Still, nobody bothered in my day. Everyone was at it. You should have heard Johny G in his heyday, pure silk and velvet on forty a day. Olivier once had a brand named after him, did you know that? I grow old, I grow old. I shall smoke my tobacco fresh-rolled. Veteran trouper takes last stand. Sorry if I'm sounding maudlin. I can hardly remember what it was like to be a student.'

'How old are you now?'

'A hundred and three . . .'

He felt it tonight. It had been a long, depressing evening. He didn't want to think about Dick Jones, or the ghastly nonentities who'd walked off with tonight's prizes. Or Natasha, with her infuriatingly offhand manner towards him, or Seymour's taste in dubious friends. Tonight his range was limited; he would only play Alceste. He stared at George with misanthropic gloom.

'Tell me about Manchester.'

He listened impassively to George's descriptions of his classes, his teachers, his fellow students. The world he discussed seemed much as Philip remembered it from his own experience (inasmuch as he could still delve into that dusty mental archive) with the exception that the kids today seemed to spend a disproportionate amount of time improvising. At least, George acknowledged slyly, hanging around with Philip had given him a good grounding in spontaneous fabrication, or, as he put it, 'telling porkies'. Well, that was what acting was all about, wasn't it? Suspension of disbelief, illusion, lying. No wonder he could wear deviousness like a second skin whenever it suited him.

At length the Scotch, the hour and the repetitive drift of the conversation did their work and he began to feel drowsy. He left the sofa to George and retired next door to bed. Despite his tiredness it took him a long time to get to sleep. When finally he drifted off it was almost light again.

He was awoken, it seemed almost immediately, by the phone ringing. He was in such a deep sleep that at first he thought he was dreaming, but the persistent tone succeeded at last in breaching unconsciousness and he rolled over, reluctantly, to answer it. The phone went dead just as he got there. He looked at his watch. It was a minute after 8 o'clock. He unleashed a string of expletives, then threw a pillow over his head in a futile attempt to shut out the suddenly intrusive morning light and noise. He didn't manage to come remotely near to dozing off again.

Five minutes later George walked in, bearing a mug of coffee.

'Didn't you hear the phone?' he asked, sounding aggrieved. 'Was ringing for ages. Woke me up and all.'

'George, stop complaining, this isn't the fucking Savoy.'

'Oh, charming! Don't choke on your coffee now, will you?'

George slammed down the mug and flounced out. Philip took a sip, and winced. It was undrinkable. He reached for the radio and turned on the *Today* programme. After five minutes of listening to a cabinet minister making excuses, he got up to run a bath.

He was lying in steaming hot water, immersed to the chin, when the phone rang again. George called out plaintively from next door for him to answer it.

'I'm in the bath!' Philip shouted back. 'Get it for me, will you?'

He covered his eyes with his flannel. It was a Monday. Not a great start to the week so far, he reflected. It probably wasn't going to get much better, either. He was out of work, at a loose end, bored. There were no women in his life. His diary was a pitiful near blank. A spot of bridge planned for Wednesday, a twice-rearranged poker game with some of his old touring crowd on Friday. Unlucky in love, lucky in cards, perhaps? Probably sod all luck anywhere, he reckoned, if recent events were anything to go by.

George appeared suddenly in the bathroom door.

'What's the matter?' Philip demanded.

'Bloke on the phone. Wants to talk to you.'

'Didn't you tell him I was in the bath?'

'Says it's urgent.'

'Who is it?'

'Dunno.'

'Well find out, George. And ask him what he wants.'

Philip sank back crossly into the water. He had a headache coming on, he didn't want to talk to anybody. He wanted to go back to bed.

'Well?' he said sharply, when George reappeared.

'It's Brendan.'

'Brendan O'Malley? What on earth does Brendan want?'

'Says it's about Seymour.'

'What about Seymour?'

'He got took ill. After you left.'

'Ill? How ill?'

'He wants to talk to you about it.'

'All right . . . pass me that towel, will you?'

Reluctantly Philip got out of the bath and dried himself. He slipped on his dressing gown and went next door. He picked up the extension by his bed.

'Philip? Sorry to have woken you. I heard you had a late night.'

Philip hardly recognized Brendan's voice. For one thing, he sounded sober.

'What's this about Seymour?'

'I'm afraid it's bad, Philip.'

'You mean he really is ill?'

'Worse than ill . . .'

There was a pause at the other end.

'I'm sorry to be the one to have to tell you this, Philip, but Seymour's dead.'

4

It had happened about an hour after Philip left Bosie Butterflys. The club was closing, and Seymour had gone upstairs with Doris and Norman for a last farewell drink. He had just finished his brandy when he had a heart attack and collapsed. An ambulance arrived promptly, but attempts to revive him proved futile. He was pronounced dead on arrival at hospital.

Philip was stunned. He had known Seymour for over twenty-five years, more than half his life. Seymour had been one of the first older actors to befriend him; Philip had loved just to sit and hear him gossip, dissecting the world with his acid wit and scattering reputations like dust. But there'd always been a twinkle in the eye, the malice was leavened with outrageous good humour. Furthermore, Seymour's opinions had usually been right. He had possessed a fund of sense and had been good company personified.

> The weight of this sad time we must obey;
> Speak what we feel, not what we ought to say.
> The oldest hath borne most: we that are young,
> Shall never see so much, nor live so long.

Philip stood alone in his living room, thinking lines of remembrance, while Verdi's *Requiem* issued powerfully from the gramophone. George had been dispatched the

42

minute he'd finished speaking to Brendan; he wanted to be alone. The sense of general gloom which had weighed on him since yesterday had become all enveloping. He stared blankly out of the window.

Seymour was dead.

He took it in, but couldn't take it in. He'd never known anyone as vital as Seymour; he had brimmed with life. He was seventy-two, Brendan had told him by way of explanation, and that had been a shock. He had never thought of Seymour as being of pensionable age; it had never occurred to him to think his age an issue. He was like some old cruise liner, a little rusty in the bows perhaps, but forever and indomitably ploughing on. Why should he have stopped? Seventy-two wasn't old. Death wasn't in the script.

> No, no, he is dead;
> Go to thy death-bed,
> He never will come again.

He'd said his doctor had told him to go easy. He shouldn't be drinking, he said, but Philip had let him. Philip had scoffed at his gloomy talk. He felt responsible.

It was ridiculous, he knew, but still he couldn't shake off that twinge of guilt. No man could tell his hour, a glass less of semi-alcoholic lemonade wasn't going to keep the old sickle bearer on hold for long. If your heart wasn't up to it you could just go any moment, like that, snap!

Philip's hand trembled as he lit a cigarette. He smoked far too much; drank like a fish; didn't exercise enough. He'd always been naturally slim, but his waistbands were getting suspiciously tight and he was labouring for breath just coming up the stairs. He was getting on, the big Five-O loomed. He'd better start taking care of himself.

He stubbed out the cigarette, put on his coat and set off for a brisk walk across Highbury Fields. A spot of exercise to get the circulation going. He went past the swimming pool, made a mental note to use it more regularly. Perhaps he'd even have to start thinking about visiting a gym, a notion he'd always dreaded. He'd contemplate anything, within reason, which meant anything except jogging. If it was a toss-up between jogging and death he'd choose death.

He carried on along Upper Street and popped into his local bookshop, where he bought three diet books and a thick volume purporting to offer near immortality and a quack-free existence. He crossed the road to the supermarket in a state of hyper-paranoia and came out laden with quantities of fruit and green vegetables. Knowing his luck, he'd probably peg out with a vitamin overdose.

His answerphone machine was blinking at him when he got home. The suave-sounding man on the message announced that he was Nigel Loseby and that his father's funeral service would be held on Friday at the Actors' Church in Covent Garden, followed by interment in the Brompton Cemetery. He trusted that Philip, as one of his father's oldest friends, would be free to attend, and hoped that he could be prevailed upon to speak a few words. He left a number at the Ministry where he could be reached.

Philip rang back at once and spoke to Loseby's secretary. Of course he would be at the service, and he would be honoured to deliver the peroration. He offered his sympathies for Nigel's sad loss. He replaced Verdi with Mahler, took pen and paper, and began to compose.

He spent most of the week working on his speech. It wasn't enough, the words still sounded hollow as he ran through them in the back of the taxi on the way to church. He might have to extemporize, though the thought of going in without a finished script made him uncomfortable. Seymour's farewell would be a command performance before a star-studded congregation.

They were gathering on the pavement as his taxi drew

up. He nodded solemnly, catching the eyes of knights and dames, and just managing to conceal his surprise at the sight of more than one old trouper whom he had thought long consigned to the grave ahead of Seymour. He tilted his profile discreetly to catch the flashes of the press photographers and stopped, with head bowed and a suitable expression, just perfectly in shot for the TV camera mounted on the church steps. A reporter was interviewing one of the country's most distinguished actors.

'. . . a terrible loss,' the great titled thespian intoned. 'He was a wonderful, lovely man, it's very sad. Today we're saying goodbye not just to a man; we're tearing out a page of theatrical history.'

Bugger! thought Philip crossly. He'd been going to say just that in his own speech.

'And he was of course wickedly witty as well as fantastically generous. You know what Ralph Richardson once said of him?'

'Of course I bloody do,' Philip answered under his breath. 'I was going to say that too, you garrulous beknighted twit!'

Philip mounted the steps to the church in a huff. He'd have to get a quiet moment behind a pillar to go over his lines.

But quiet moments inside would be hard to come by; the interior was awash with friends and acquaintances. Brendan was there, and Lindsay, Maggie, Tony, Jack, Bob. It was even whispered that darling Johny might put in an appearance. If someone had exploded a bomb in the nave, Shaftesbury Avenue and the South Bank would have had to shut up shop for the duration.

'Well, Philip,' said Brendan O'Malley ruefully, 'I never thought it'd come to this. I was convinced old Loseby would see us all out.'

'I know. I said as much to him the night he died. It's been a terrible shock.'

45

'Just what exactly were you doing with him in Bosie Butterflys, Philip? Finding a heterosexual in that dump is like meeting a rabbi in Mecca.'

'I'm surprised I didn't see you there, Brendan.'

'Can't stand the place. S&M's not my scene and the sight of that fat old queen who runs it makes me want to retch. Don't say it takes one to know one.'

'Would I stoop so low?'

'You'd be well advised not to in Bosie Butterflys. I suppose we'd better raise the tone of the conversation. Good morning to you, Vicar!'

The vicar wanted to talk to Philip about the service. Apparently Seymour had left detailed instructions. An actor to the last, it was clearly his intention to back out of the limelight only with the greatest reluctance. Philip was offered a seat in the centre front row, just below the specially sited lectern. He might have preferred to mount the pulpit, stage right and suitably imposing, but he supposed that the designated position offered greater informality. He took his seat and studied his notes.

The organ started up. Expecting something solemn, he was startled to hear the jaunty, familiar tune. He turned round in his seat, and found that everybody else was turning round in theirs, hoping to catch a confirmatory eye. The rows of grave faces lightened and a general smile spread across the congregation. Yes, the organist really was playing 'Oh, I do like to be beside the seaside!'.

'Dear Seymour,' Philip murmured to Lindsay Leonard, who was just settling in beside him. 'I'll miss the old bugger.'

Lindsay smiled wanly, and brushed back a theatrical tear. There would be a few of those flowing today, Philip reflected. He glanced around, and saw all necks craning towards the entrance. Nigel Loseby had just entered, and was proceeding down the aisle, followed by an equine bleached-blonde wife and two small sour-faced reluctant children. It looked like the kind of family most politicians would be anxious to spend less time with, though Philip, as a rabid bachelor, would have had to concede that he was not best placed to judge. The Losebys took the front pew opposite his own. Philip smiled at them sympathetically. Young Nigel reciprocated, then responded with a nod to the vicar's signal. The ceremony was about to begin.

The organist made a fluent change of tack and, to the accompaniment of The Dead March from Saul, four strapping pallbearers (and they needed to be) made their dignified entrance. So often the supporting player, Seymour would have revelled in the moment. It was all Philip could do to prevent himself from rising and applauding.

'Let us pray,' said the vicar, and the whole godless crew of veteran theatricals, adulterers, fornicators, sodomites, supreme blasphemers, and, in one case at least, conscienceless murderers, sank to their knees in a faultless synchronized display of freestyle humility.

Afterwards they sang 'Onward Christian Soldiers' and 'All Things Bright and Beautiful' (complete with all politically incorrect verses; Seymour was a stickler for detail) and listened to Lindsay reading Shakespeare's most glorious song.

> Fear no more the heat o' the sun,
>   Nor the furious winter's rages;
> Thou thy worldly task hast done,
>   Home art gone, and ta'en thy wages;
> Golden lads and girls all must,
> As chimney-sweepers, come to dust.

None listened more intently than Philip, who was relieved to discover that the acoustic wasn't half bad. When she had finished, the vicar took the lectern and delivered himself of a few ill-informed words, concluding, in reference to the four Losebys present, with a comical tribute to

Seymour's unshakeable faith in the virtues of family life. After a few more prayers he stepped down. It was Philip's cue.

He walked up slowly to the lectern. He could afford to take his time; every eye was on him. He put on his glasses, laid down his notes, and peered at them carefully for a count of five. Philip didn't actually wear glasses, but they were the best prop in the world for suggesting thoughtful gravitas, and he had several clear-lensed pairs ready for such occasions. Once he'd gone through the motions of preparing himself, of course, he took them off again. He didn't want to obscure his face.

'Seymour Loseby was more than a friend. Seymour Loseby was more than an actor. This was a man. We shall not see his like again.'

He paused to measure his voice. Right tone – perhaps half a notch up on the volume. He made the necessary adjustment.

'I first met Seymour in the early 1960s, in Windsor. Rattigan, Lonsdale, Barrie, were in the repertory. The Experimental Theatre Season, Seymour called it. "This is a famous old theatre, you know," he told me on the first day of rehearsals. "I should warn you – at Windsor the queen is *always* in residence." It was a riotous time; I've never heard so much laughter in a green room, and the cause was Seymour. It was impossible to be pompous in his presence, his good humour was infectious and disarming; the bubble reputation can rarely have been so often pricked, and never with such absence of malice. In all my own experience as an actor, nothing has ever quite matched the thrill of discovering, on the first day of rehearsals, that Seymour was in the cast. It was like finding out that you had David Gower coming in to bat for you, first wicket down. As a lover of good cricket, or more especially, good cricketers, I trust he would have approved of the analogy.'

Philip paused to enjoy the knowing smiles of Seymour's more louche friends in the congregation. As he didn't have any unlouche friends, this meant practically everyone. Seymour had been famously indifferent to the sport of cricket, but the sight of athletic young men in crisp white flannels had been enough, by his own admission, to drive him into a sexual frenzy. He maintained that one of the most attractive aspects of touring was the chance it gave him to hang around country pavilions on a Sunday afternoon. A sniff of linseed oil would send him into transports of delight.

But these were not the kind of details Philip supposed the Loseby heirs would wish to hear. He dwelt instead on the man's personal and professional qualities, omitting by graceful elision or shading with recondite code those episodes unfit for general consumption. It was a sophisticated audience. No implication was left undrawn, no hint unsavoured. Seymour would have loved it.

'A chatterbox, an incurable gossip? Yes, by his own admission. His candour was irrepressible. He loved to quote Tallulah Bankhead: "Talk badly of me if you must, talk well of me if you can, but for heaven's sake talk about me." I can only speak well of him, and I speak for all of us here, too. He would have loved today. I remember him once being upbraided for turning up to rehearsal five minutes in arrears with the charge that he would be late for his own funeral. Seymour was stunned. "But my dear," he answered the director with astonishment. "Everyone will be talking about me. I might miss something!" The only people missing something today are we, his friends. He would not mind me saying that he was larger than life. "I'm a talented linguist," I once heard him declare backstage at the National Theatre, to a bemused gathering of distinguished international actors. "I speak fluent Cliché." He had Falstaff's presence, and Mercutio's wit. It is our consolation that he who was larger than life is much,

49

much larger than death. We will always remember him, not least because it will be impossible to forget him. The other day, as I was looking through my own mementoes and scrapbooks, I came across a card he sent me at the close of some long-forgotten play – a typically perverse gesture, one might think, to send a last-night and not a first-night greeting. There was a verse of Thackeray's written out in his own hand:

> The play is done; the curtain drops,
>   Slow falling to the prompter's bell:
> A moment yet the actor stops,
>   And looks around, to say farewell.
> It is an irksome word and task:
>   And, when he's laughed, and said his say,
> He shows, as he removes the mask,
>   A face that's anything but gay.

'The last line was underscored heavily in purple ink and finished with exclamation marks. Seymour had added underneath, simply, "Who said the age of innocence was dead?"

'It is in part to mourn the passing of another age that we are here today. It is a humbling experience to stand in this beautiful old church, to look at the plaques on the wall, to read the illustrious names of so many who have adorned our profession. Today I have been reminded of some who, half a century ago, inducted the young Seymour Loseby into the theatrical mysteries. Their personalities, their performances, are vivid in my imagination because Seymour and others of his generation have made them live for me. So too will he live for as long as we have breath to commemorate him. The baton is passed on, the curtain comes down only to rise again, the show goes on. I trust that Seymour would have approved my hackneyed fluency. If he didn't, he'd have been sure to let me know.

As he once remarked to me when I was struggling with a part, with an avuncular pat on the shoulder, "If at first you don't succeed, Philip, for God's sake give up." We, his friends, must be grateful that he never followed his own advice. We shall miss him.'

Philip paused at the lectern long enough to collect his notes and savour the oddly gratifying silence. Applause, of course, was not to be expected, but he sensed an undercurrent of approbation. Lindsay took his hand as he resumed his pew and whispered a heartfelt, 'Well done,' in his ear.

The vicar reassumed his centre-stage role and enjoined them all to rise for the singing of 'Jerusalem'. Afterwards they knelt for a few final prayers and then stood in solemn silence as the coffin was lifted on to the shoulders of the pallbearers. As they began their measured procession, the organist broke out into a spirited rendition of 'All the nice girls love a sailor' and the solemnity was in an instant dissipated. The service ended much as it had begun, with the majority of the congregation attempting to control their smiles.

There was laughter all the way to the cemetery too, in the back of the cab Philip was sharing with Brendan, Lindsay and Denis, a sometime theatrical dresser who had done up zips and buttons for them all and was nowadays working for one of the top firms of costumiers. Denis, in particular, was full of tales of Seymour which Philip had never heard. Their friend had lived life to the full, and then some.

They were among the first to arrive at the cemetery, one of the most beautiful in London and, according to Brendan and Denis, a great place to go cruising. As a lot of actors were buried there Seymour should feel doubly at home, they reckoned. He was destined for the Loseby family plot in the southwestern corner, distressingly near the ugly pile of Chelsea football ground. While waiting for the cortege to arrive, Philip took a quiet wander round. He was reading

51

the inscriptions on some Victorian tombstones when Nigel Loseby came and found him.

'We've got a couple of minutes,' said the politician quietly. 'Mind if we talk?'

'Not at all.'

Philip shrugged. He indicated the path. The two of them set off along it at a slow pace. Nigel's minder, a compact heavy in a thick dark overcoat, followed at a discreet distance.

'Must be a bore,' Philip commented. 'The security.'

'You get used to it. I forget he's there after a while. Thank you for delivering the address.'

'I was honoured to be asked. We were very old friends.'

'Of course. It came out in what you said. I hadn't realized you'd known him for quite so long. Look, I'm sorry to have to ask you this, it's . . . it's a little delicate.'

Nigel Loseby stopped and tore off a stalk of the unkempt waist-high grass. Philip watched him twist it round his finger in a deft, elaborate gesture reminiscent of his father. The boy didn't look at all like him (angular and dark, as opposed to round and fair), but there was an occasional echo of Seymour's expansiveness in his manner, a hint of the baroque to lighten the plain Gothic construction that was the junior minister. Seymour had had nothing to do with the boy's upbringing, indeed had hardly known his son during the first three decades of his life, but something must have rubbed off in the last few years. Seymour had been pleasantly surprised at how fond he'd become of the young man to whom he had referred for so long as, '*Ma folie de boudoir*'.

'My father,' Nigel continued awkwardly, 'was not, in many ways, a conventional man.'

Not in any way at all, Philip thought to himself. He smiled politely. Nigel finished tearing his stalk of grass to shreds.

'I don't know if you saw any of the papers after his death.'

'I read all the obituaries.'

'No, I don't mean that – very kind they were, though, I was pleased. No, I'm talking about the tabloids. Just one of them, actually, but there was a bit of innuendo, it was all rather tacky, left a nasty taste in the mouth.'

'Can you expect anything else from the tabloids.'

'Yes, you're right. I suppose I should be relieved that there wasn't anything more to it – '

'What was there exactly?'

'Oh, just a line or two about that club where he died, saying it had a bit of a "reputation". Nothing more explicit than that. Snide, though, I thought.'

'If that's all there was to it I think you're being a mite oversensitive.'

'I wish I could agree with you. I've had dealings with these muckraking journalists before. If there's anything they can dig up on my father they'll use it against me without a second thought.'

'I can see they might throw some mud, but it wouldn't stick, surely? Seymour liked to hang around gay bars and preferred the company of men who wore earrings. So what? We don't get to choose our own parents. No one can hold you responsible.'

'Not in the world you inhabit, no. Politics is rather different.'

'If the scandals that have been hitting the papers recently are anything to go by, politics is rather worse.'

'Which is precisely why I'm worried.'

'You mean your career wouldn't stand any aftershock?'

'Look, I realize I may sound unduly mercenary, hypocritical, even, but the fact is I am ambitious – I make no bones about it and I wouldn't expect you, as an actor, to either – and I can't afford to have too unorthodox a set of family values paraded before the *Sun*-reading public for their prurient consumption in the weeks leading up to what is likely to be the most major cabinet reshuffle of the present term.'

'I can understand that, but what exactly do you want from me?'

'I just would be very grateful if you didn't speak to the papers, that's all. What you said in church today is all right for friends and fellow theatricals, but I shouldn't like to read it in black and white over my Sunday breakfast.'

'Ah. I see.'

They had completed a small circuit of the corner of the cemetery. At the end of the path they could see the hearse just turning in. Nigel's wife detached herself from the crowd by the graveside and came towards them.

'Since you've been so frank with me I'll be frank with you,' Philip told him quietly, while nodding politely to his approaching other half. 'I don't think much of your timing, but we'll let that pass. I've no intention of speaking to anyone, the thought hadn't even crossed my mind. I hope that satisfies you, although I do have to say I don't think I'm really your problem. There may be some decidedly odd worms in the woodwork, and there's not a lot any of us can do about them. I shall keep my fingers crossed for you, however, and hope that you emerge unscathed with a suitably enlarged portfolio by the end of the summer. Your father would have wanted that very much. And now I think you'd better introduce me to your charming wife . . .'

The charm was little in evidence during their brief encounter. The Losebys' marriage, Philip decided, operated under conditions of polite strain. At the end of the brief but impressive graveside ceremony he declined the general invitation to join them for refreshments at their house in Hollywood Road. Instead he and Brendan took a cab back to Soho and had a commemorative drink (Philip's was soft, to Brendan's astonishment) in Seymour's favourite pub.

54

Philip did not get back home again until the late afternoon, whereupon he encountered two surprises.

The first surprise was a large brown paper package that was waiting for him in the hallway, so bulky he could hardly get it up the stairs. It turned out to be an exercise bicycle, ordered only three days previously and delivered with uncharacteristic efficiency.

The second surprise was his discovery of a message from Nigel Loseby on the answerphone. The junior minister sounded agitated. He left his Chelsea number and begged Philip to phone him the moment he got in. Philip had only seen him a few hours ago. What could he possibly want? He picked up the phone.

And after he had finished talking to the Rt Hon Nigel Loseby, MP, he was even more surprised.

5

Philip was cycling on his new machine when the doorbell rang an hour later. It had taken him most of that time to get the damned thing assembled. He dismounted reluctantly at the second buzz and noticed with some alarm that he had just travelled all of four hundred yards. He felt like he'd finished a leg of the Tour de France.

'First floor,' he panted into the intercom as he released the button. He opened the door, walked over to the window and peered out. A substantial official black car was sitting outside, with a uniformed chauffeur at the wheel. It would be rather fine to have one of those, he decided, and pictured himself cruising down Shaftesbury Avenue and alighting in a welter of envy and admiration on the steps of the Garrick Club. Unfortunately he'd only been on the waiting list for three years. By the time they got round to admitting him he'd be travelling by hearse, not limousine.

'Can I offer you anything?' he asked young Loseby as he appeared in the doorway. 'Tea? Coffee? Alcohol?'

'No, thank you,' the junior minister replied tersely. He stood just over the threshold, his coat buttoned up and his hands thrust into his pockets. Under his coat he was wearing a dinner jacket. 'I can't stay too long.'

'Well, you'll have to excuse me while I fix something for myself,' said Philip pleasantly, adding (by way of explanation as he went into the kitchen): 'I've been exercising!'

He opened the fridge and examined the cartons on the

top shelf. He chose a pure blackcurrant juice with added extra minerals. He returned to the living room and saw that Nigel Loseby was still standing by the door.

'Please,' he said, indicating the sofa.

Nigel sat down reluctantly. He fumbled in his pocket for cigarettes and offered Philip the packet.

'No, thanks, I've given up,' said Philip, pushing an ashtray across the coffee table. He crossed to the nearest window and opened it wide.

'I'm sorry,' said Nigel, hesitating before lighting up. 'If you'd rather I didn't . . .'

'No, no,' said Philip indulgently, sitting down in his armchair. 'Please, be my guest. You *are* my guest. What you do to your lungs is your own affair! Now, as you're sitting comfortably, and if, as you say, you really can't stay long, please do tell me what this is all about. Your mysterious manner on the phone quite intrigued me.'

Nigel lit up. He glanced at the open window.

'Are you sure we can't be overheard?'

Philip, who had given no thought at all to the matter, could only look bemused.

'It's always possible that my downstairs neighbours are even now standing on a stepladder with stethoscopes pressed to the ceiling, but I shouldn't have thought it likely. You never can tell, though.'

'I'm sorry, you must think I'm being paranoid.'

'Mm . . .'

Philip sat back in his armchair and examined his visitor with keen interest. It was a familiar face, he'd seen it countless times in newspapers and on TV. Nigel Loseby was photo- and telegenic and he knew it; utter confidence was refracted through every lens. Arrogance, his opponents called it, and it certainly wasn't hard to see that he thought a lot of himself. If his voice had been a little more expressive, he might have made a good actor.

But he didn't look arrogant now. At the cemetery he

had carried a slight air of hesitancy, but somewhere in the course of the afternoon it had turned into raging uncertainty. The cameras would scarcely have recognized the pale vulnerable man sitting opposite him on the very edge of the sofa and pulling tensely on his cigarette.

'Just what exactly might you be paranoid about, Nigel?' Philip asked him, gently. 'You said on the phone that something awkward had come up, you were in trouble. What kind of trouble, and how can I possibly help? It wouldn't have anything to do with what we were talking about at the funeral, would it?'

Nigel looked shocked. During a long pause he didn't move, then suddenly the breath came whistling out in a long sigh. He slumped back on the sofa, the tension pricked out of him. He seemed relieved.

'I'm sorry to involve you in this, Philip; I just don't know who else to turn to. I don't know if you can help me, but if you can't, no one can.'

'Help you with what?'

'I'm being blackmailed.'

Nigel took a drag of his half-finished cigarette, stubbed it out in the ashtray with a profligate flourish and immediately lit another. Now that he'd got it out he sounded quite calm, perhaps fatalistic.

'You're right. It's precisely what we were talking about. I just didn't expect it to blow up so soon, that's all. This man called me up about five minutes after I'd got home. That was nice.'

'What man?'

'I've no idea who he was, he didn't give a name. Not surprisingly.'

'Surely you're ex-directory? How did he get your number?'

'From my father's diary.'

'His diary? Where on earth did he get hold of that?'

'That's what I'd like to know. God. Of all the things that

could have happened, this is the worst. I'm sorry, I think I'd like a drink after all.'

'Scotch?'

'Thanks. I'll take it neat, please.'

Philip filled half a tumbler and carried it over. Nigel took a heavy slug, winced, and took another.

'Sorry, I'm a bit on edge, as you can understand . . . where was I?'

'The diary.'

'Yes. Or perhaps I should say journal; I'm not sure what my father would have called it. He didn't just keep a record of appointments, though he did that too. He must have had a photographic memory, a mania for detail. Nothing was left out. Unfortunately. All the volumes – thick hardbacks, A5 size – were neatly arranged by his bedside, each one covering three or four years. There were about a dozen. I read them, it was quite a shock. Talk about explicit. Dates, places, names – by God, you should have seen some of the names! I loved my father dearly, but I'm afraid he was a terrible old pervert.'

Philip shrugged. After a lifetime in the theatre, he could spot a pervert at fifty paces in good light. With Seymour, he'd always suspected, there'd been much more talk than action. Besides, given his own sexual peccadilloes, he'd never felt inclined to pass judgement.

'Nigel, I can understand that your public position makes you sensitive, but I really must stress again that no one can hold you personally responsible for what your father got up to. It isn't the first time something like this has happened. There might be a bit of fuss, but it'll die down. So someone has got hold of one of these diaries. How? He must have stolen it. That's a serious offence. Tell him to publish and be damned, because he will be. Attempted blackmail and handling stolen goods – we're not talking about a suspended sentence and a slap on the wrist here.'

'It's too risky, Philip. Of course I'm not responsible for

my father. You know that, I know that, anyone with any intelligence knows that, but I'm not talking about intelligent and sophisticated people. I'm talking about the modern Conservative Party. My constituency chairman thinks hanging's too good for first-time parking offenders. And most of his committee think he's left wing.'

'This is a much better story than anything Seymour got up to. I might speak to the press after all.'

'I'd deny everything. But I can't deny what's in black and white in Dad's own handwriting. I can't even prove the diary was stolen, either. It's the final volume, you see. The last one by his bedside stops four years ago. It wasn't taken from his flat. He must have had it on him when he died. Whoever's got it could claim he gave it to them. Of course, he didn't, but who can predict what a jury might say? Not that I'm prepared to argue it out in court – remember the Fiona Wright case? It's no damned good me being technically in the right, you know. Can you imagine the sleaze there'd be in the papers? Forget the legal niceties, he's got me by the balls.'

'How much does he want?'

'A hundred and fifty thousand pounds.'

'That's ridiculous!'

'I know. I tried to negotiate.'

'What did you offer?'

'I didn't get round to offering anything. He put the phone down on me. What do you think it's worth?'

'Whatever he'd get from a Sunday tabloid. Difficult to say without having seen the material myself, but if we're talking about bringing down a member of the government I'm afraid we're not talking peanuts.'

'I was afraid you'd say that. I haven't got very much money.'

'Given your address and lifestyle, the blackmailer might find that hard to credit.'

'I know, but it's true. Everything I've got's tied up,

mostly in the mortgage. A junior minister's salary isn't much. I'm already living beyond my means. I've made some unfortunate investments. Lloyd's, you know . . .'

'How much can you afford?'

'Ready cash? Ten, maybe. I'm not quite sure. Given time I can raise a bit more, but nothing remotely close to a hundred and fifty thousand.'

'Your blackmailer's not going to like that.'

'I know. But if I could lean on him a bit, if I could bluff him – something along the lines you were suggesting, threatening to involve the police (God knows I wouldn't, but could he be sure?), I might, I just might be able to knock him down to a reasonable figure. The only problem is that I don't know who this man is. While I have to wait for him to call me, while I'm reduced to a nervous wreck waiting for the phone to ring, he's got the upper hand. But if I could find out who he is, if I could get the bastard face to face on my terms, that might unnerve him.'

'You might just panic him into selling out to the first hack he speaks to. On the other hand, you might be right.'

'It's worth finding out. I mean, I can't pay what he's asking, so I couldn't be any worse off, could I? Look, it's one thing to make anonymous threats, another to back them up in the flesh. Blackmailing's a pretty low-down cowardly occupation, even by criminal standards, maybe this chap'll crack if I can put the spotlight on him. Which brings me back to my big problem. Just who the hell is he? That's where I'm hoping you can help me.'

'You think I'm the type who consorts with low-down criminals?'

'No, but you were with my father the night he died. You know who was there, the kind of people he hung around with. Somehow I don't think they're heroes, Philip. Dad said you were the most resourceful man he knew, he said you always had your ear to the ground. You might even recognize the blackmailer's voice. You see, I've got it on tape.'

Nigel reached into his inside coat pocket and took out a black mini-cassette recorder. He laid it down on the coffee table.

'It's perhaps just as well that I am paranoid, Philip. You get that way in politics. I've been so blatantly misquoted so often that I take the precaution of recording every telephone conversation I have.'

'Good. Let's hear it.'

It wasn't a long conversation. It began with a light but gruff voice demanding to speak to the master of the house. 'I've got something that might interest you,' it went on when Nigel had identified himself, 'something that belonged to daddy. He was a naughty boy, was daddy . . .' The tone of the voice was arch, insinuating, and very sure of itself. Somehow Philip doubted that its owner would be easily intimidated.

It referred to the diary as 'daddy's address book, with some spicy undressed bits in it', and suggested that the readers of one particular downmarket weekend paper might be tickled to peruse its contents over their Sunday cornflakes. Should Nigel wish to prevent this unfortunate occurrence, he would have to cough up a hundred and fifty K in used notes with nothing above a twenty. When Nigel cut in to protest the voice answered sharply that the fee was not negotiable and warned him to have it ready by the same time tomorrow night, when he would be rung up and told where to take it. At that point the conversation ended.

'There was a bit more, but it didn't record properly,' Nigel explained, pressing the rewind button. 'It's enough, though, isn't it? Does it mean anything to you?'

'I'm afraid not,' replied Philip smoothly. 'Would you mind playing it again, though, just in case.'

Nigel looked despondent, but he did as he was told.

Philip got up and walked slowly over to the window. He was only half listening to the tape. He was thinking.

'Sorry, no,' he repeated with a pained expression, when the tape had run. He shook his head sadly. 'That voice is unknown to me.'

Nigel crumpled up a little further. He muttered something inaudible and went to light another cigarette. Philip chose his moment carefully.

'On the other hand . . .'

Nigel glanced up.

'I just might – only might – be able to help.'

Nigel sat staring at him intently, his unfired lighter pressed to the tip of his cigarette. Philip had him on tenterhooks. He let him hang there. Without hurrying, he resumed his seat.

'How?' Nigel demanded at length in a hoarse voice, when he could no longer bear waiting for Philip to settle himself down.

Again, Philip took his time before replying. He had his audience where he wanted it and actors, like confidence tricksters, need their customers to come on to them. At that moment he could have sold him anything.

'As you so rightly surmised, I am familiar with your father's milieu. I don't know the voice on the tape, but I may know a man who does. In that case, I might be able to get myself into a position where I could exert a little appropriate leverage. Of course, it could be dangerous.'

'Dangerous?'

'It's a closed world, prying strangers aren't welcome. Somebody thinks he can make a lot of money out of that diary. The stakes are high.'

'But . . . I can't have you exposing yourself to any danger –'

'I can take care of myself, Nigel. As your father noted, I am not unresourceful. And sometimes you just have to be prepared to run a few risks – if, that is, the reward is right . . .'

Philip sat back in his chair, keeping his eyes locked firmly on to Nigel's. His own expression was cool and business-like. He wanted to be sure that Nigel understood him. Nigel did.

'As I say, Philip, I'm not a rich man. Of course, I'd be extremely grateful, and no doubt we might be able to come to some small financial arrangement, but –'

'I'm not talking about money,' Philip interrupted crisply. 'As you've just explained, you don't have any. No, I have something else in mind. Like you, I'm ambitious. It's a vice you yourself have admitted to freely; I return your candour. I too have my plans. Now, if yours come to fruition, as you hope and all the commentators seem to expect, then after this next cabinet reshuffle you should find yourself in a position of no mean influence. If, that is, we can keep the lid on Seymour's squalid little adventures. I should then have done the state some service. I should like the state to bear that in mind when the next New Year's Honours List comes up for discussion.'

'Philip, the Honours List isn't a party political matter –'

'Oh come, come, dear boy! What was the average contri-bution of new life peers to party funds during the eighties? Two hundred grand, wasn't it? And cheap at the price, too; Lloyd George got a much better deal. I may be biased, but I think I'm a much more deserving case. I've put in a lot of damned hard donkey work over the years for the greater glory of the British theatre. To tell you the truth, I'm feeling rather miffed that I've been overlooked thus far.'

'Well, of course, you're a very distinguished actor, one of our very finest, dare I say . . . Yes, I'd fully agree, you're probably overdue for an MBE –'

'Bugger that, dear, it's the full works I'm after. I want to be able to get a decent table in restaurants.'

'You don't mean – a knighthood?'

'The very same. Sir Philip Fletcher. Trips off the tongue, eh?'

It didn't look like it was going to trip off Nigel's tongue. For a long half-minute he stared at Philip dumbly, his eyes wide open with amazement. Philip occupied the interlude dreaming pleasantly of the gala opening of the newly rechristened Sir Philip Fletcher Auditorium at the Royal National Theatre.

'You don't beat about the bush, do you?' Nigel commented grimly at last. 'Let me get this straight. You'll help me out if I get you a knighthood? What if I can't?'

'I'm a busy man, Nigel. Alas, there are many demands on my time.'

'So you won't help me unless I help you? You want to blackmail me too?'

'It's hardly the same thing.'

'Really? You'll have to forgive me if I don't quite see it that way. Here am I over a barrel, I'm turning to my father's oldest and dearest friend as my last hope in an impossible situation, only to find you too putting the squeeze on me, making ridiculous demands which I'm in no position to fulfil. It's downright immoral!'

'To you and me, maybe, but what's downright immoral to your constituents, alas, is the contents of daddy's diary. All I'm asking for is a small token of recognition in return for keeping them out of the public domain. I'm quite offended that you're making such a fuss. Ridiculous demands, indeed! If a worthless talentless scumbag like Dick Jones can get a handle, I see no reason on earth why I shouldn't have one too.'

'Dick Jones? How on earth did you know . . . ? Oh God. Oh, don't tell me . . .'

'I'm afraid so, Nigel. It really wasn't a very good idea to confide in your father. He had many estimable qualities, but discretion was not amongst them. Dick Jones, on the other hand, has no estimable qualities whatsoever, and his imminent elevation to the ranks of the great and the good is an abomination of the first order. What can the Prime Minister have been thinking of?'

'I know,' murmured Nigel glumly, 'he's got no taste.'

'Whereas you, on the other hand, have it to spare. As one of the few prominent politicians of any party within living memory to appreciate the difference between King Lear and King Kong, and given the authority conveyed upon you by your estimable family theatrical connections, I should think you ideally placed to drop a quiet word of recommendation into the right ear at the appropriate moment. I know the way these things work, and I know how well connected you are. If faced with a choice between coughing up a cool one hundred and fifty K which you haven't got; or enduring massive and career-terminating public humiliation; or simply arranging for little old me to get a modest invite to meet HM At Home, I know which I'd go for. But please, don't let me influence you in any way . . .'

Nigel sat staring distractedly at the carpet. He went to light another cigarette, then realized that he still had the last one smouldering in the ashtray. He picked up his glass and put it to his lips, only to discover that it was empty. Philip obliged him with a refill.

'I'd better go easy,' Nigel said, glancing at his watch. He looked surprised. 'Good God! Is that the time? I'm late, I've got to go.'

He stuffed his cigarettes and lighter into his pocket and got up, buttoning his coat. He reached for the black mini-cassette recorder.

'I'd quite like to borrow that,' said Philip. 'That is, if you still think you might like to use my services.'

Nigel stopped in the act of putting the recorder away.

'What exactly do you propose to do, Philip?'

'Why, attempt to recover the diary.'

'How?'

'I'm afraid you'll have to leave the details to me. You'll need to do some sums and let me know how much precisely you can afford to pay. He said he'd ring again tomorrow night. Screen your phone calls, don't talk to him before then. I'll speak to you first.'

'You think you'll have got somewhere by tomorrow?'

'Time, as they say, is of the essence. I'll get cracking right away. That is, if you want me to. All I'm asking for in return – and I really don't think it's very much – is your intercession in the little matter we have discussed. And please, you must understand, I'm not asking for this favour merely on my own account. If you can secure my elevation to offset the absurd and unmerited promotion of the unspeakable Jones, the entire British theatre will be eternally grateful to you.'

'You don't sell yourself short, do you?'

'There are enough people in my profession trying to do that for me already. I expect you have the same problem. Politics and the theatre have a lot in common.'

'So my father always said . . .'

Nigel looked down at the tape recorder in his hand. He seemed literally to be weighing it up. After a few moments he put it back down on the table, as Philip had known that he would. Nonetheless, he permitted himself an inward satisfied sigh. It was as good as a signature on a contract.

'If you think it'll help . . .' Nigel gave him an imploring look. 'I'm sunk if any of this comes out. You'll be discreet?'

'If I'm not I'll only be harming my own case. If you do sink I'll never get my just deserts.'

'Philip, I can't promise anything –'

'Nothing at all?'

'Well, I can promise to do my best, that's –'

'That's enough, Nigel. I have faith in you. I think you usually get what you want. Now, you'd better get going, or you really will be late.'

Philip walked him to the door.

'Anywhere interesting you're off to?' he asked pleasantly.

'Fundraising dinner. Young Conservatives.'

'Sooner you than me. Don't choke on the rubber chicken. I'll give you a call as soon as I know anything.'

Philip saw him out. When Nigel had gone, he picked up the mini-cassette recorder and crossed over to the window. He rewound the tape and listened to it again while watching the chauffeur-driven car disappear off towards Highbury Corner. He switched off the machine and casually tossed it into an armchair.

He had recognized the voice instantly. He'd been half expecting it anyway, all things considered, but a couple of choice drawled vowels had been enough to confirm his suspicions. The voice was unmistakable. Nigel's blackmailer was none other than Doris Afternoon, queen of the Bosie Butterflys cabaret.

'Naughty, naughty, Doris!' he murmured reprovingly, sorting through the rack of CDs on his sideboard. He picked out one given as a present by his aunt Marjorie, and to which he had never listened, entitled the 'Coronation Collection'. It sounded suitably regal. He turned up the volume, fell back into his armchair, and let the opening bars of 'Zadok the Priest' fan the conflagration in his veins.

He spent an exquisite half-hour in fantasy land, dreaming details of his appointment at the Palace and his wonderfully witty conversation with the Queen; swimming in the flow of all the homage, supplication and devotion that would inevitably follow his transfiguration; and, simply, bathing in the glow of his own ineffable grandeur.

6

It was just after ten o'clock the next morning when Philip turned off Tottenham Court Road and began to thread his way through the crossroad puzzle of small streets that lies between Soho and the Marylebone Road. He passed a familiar restaurant and a redbrick mansion block where someone or other had lived twenty years ago, but it was not an area he knew well and he had to consult the A–Z in the back of his Filofax several times before he could locate the exact street he wanted. It all looked very different by daylight, of course. Without its neon halo, the entrance to the club was easily missable.

He descended the basement steps and found that the door was locked. He pressed the intercom, and after a moment heard it crackle. A rasping voice cut in before he could speak.

'Wait in the lobby with the others till you're called.'

There was a long buzz and the door clicked. Feeling somewhat bemused, Philip stepped inside.

Three female impersonators were sitting in a row beneath the portrait of Lord Alfred Douglas. Philip supposed that they must have been almost as surprised to see him as he was to see them.

'Look what the cat brought in!' said the one in the middle, who was dressed in red with a lot of black-lace frills. Three sets of eyelashes to a combined length of at least fifty metres fluttered at him in unison.

'I think he looks better in tights,' suggested one of the others coyly.

Philip was flattered. It was always nice to be recognized, whatever the circumstances. One of the things that really made an actor's life worthwhile was being whispered about, winked over and pointed at in public, no matter how much he might attempt to deny it. Philip, to his credit, never did.

'Why, thank you, ladies,' he said with gallantry. 'Perhaps you can help me. I'm looking for someone.'

'Oh, so am I,' replied the third impersonator wistfully. 'Mr Right . . .'

There was a collective sigh of sympathy from all concerned. Philip smiled kindly at each of the heavily powdered faces in turn. A nicer trio of drag queens one couldn't hope to meet.

'Actually, I'm looking for Doris Afternoon,' he explained.

'You'll be lucky!' said the one in the middle with a snort. 'She's unlikely to surface before lunch-time. How'd you think she got her name?'

The others nodded their agreement. Philip shrugged. It was exactly as Brendan had told him. Doris was a nightbird, possessed of a near-Transylvanian abhorrence of daylight. Mornings were easily the worst time to try and catch him, which was of course precisely why Philip had come.

'Conchita!' a distant voice called out from somewhere within the bowels of the building. 'Conchita de Los Angeles!'

'Ooh 'eck!' said the one in the middle, snapping open a powder compact and shooting himself a quick glance full of critical despair: 'I'm on!'

'Good luck, dear,' said one of his companions.

'Break a leg!' encouraged the other.

He probably will in those shoes, thought Philip. Conchita

tottered unsteadily for a moment, then clutched at Philip for support.

'Hold this a sec, will you?'

Philip took Conchita's silk fan, while its owner straightened the seams of his stockings.

'Don't look, saucy!'

Philip hadn't been.

'Conchita!' yelled the voice from downstairs. 'Where are you, you dozy tart?'

'Charming!' muttered Conchita crossly. Philip handed back the fan. He nodded pleasantly towards the others.

'Delighted to make your acquaintance,' he said before turning to Conchita. 'I shall accompany you down, if you don't mind.'

'Oh, don't mind me!' came the wounded reply. 'No one else does . . .'

Conchita began the long, dangerous descent of the stairs. Philip noticed a piece of paper stuck over the top of the banister with a red-inked arrow pointing downwards. The familiar legend in black above read 'AUDITIONS'.

'Nervous?' Philip enquired sympathetically.

'Bit,' answered Conchita, who was slipping down the stairs sideways, as if on skis. 'Been here before. Helps.'

'Nothing like a bit of experience, eh?'

'Oh, they're always auditioning for Bosie Butterflys. They go through acts like Warren Beatty goes through women. If only . . .'

Conchita stopped before taking the next stair and gave Philip a doe-eyed pathetic look, while whispering:

'That Norman, he's a real bastard, you know.'

'They all are, dear, it goes with the territory. Here, allow me.'

They were approaching the bottom of the staircase, which opened out and inclined to the left. Philip went ahead and offered his hand.

'Why, thank you!' said Conchita with a flush. 'You're a real gent.'

Philip inclined his head modestly.

'At bleeding last!' said a thin needling voice from the other end of the room. 'What you gonna sing for us today then, Conchita – "Slow Boat to Sodding China"?'

Norman was standing at the far end of the room by the piano. When he saw that Conchita was not alone, his naturally suspicious slitted eyes became even more weaselly.

'Who the fuck are you?'

Warmed by the greeting, Philip took his time before replying. He walked into the middle of the room, remembering sadly the occasion of his last visit, and noting how gaudy and besmirched the fittings appeared under white light. Two of the staff were behind the bar cleaning glasses.

' 'Morning, Sandy,' said Philip.

' 'Morning, Mr Fletcher,' the waiter replied. ' 'Morning, Conchita.'

'How come everyone fucking knows everyone else except for me, then?' demanded Norman sourly.

'Perhaps you should brush up your social skills,' Philip suggested. 'I've come to see Doris Afternoon.'

'You'll be lucky.'

'So I've been told. Nonetheless, would you please be so good as to pass on the message that Philip Fletcher needs to talk urgently.'

'Philip Fletcher . . . You're Seymour's friend, right?'

'I was honoured to consider myself such, yes. It is in relation to the tragic circumstances surrounding his death that I find myself here this morning.'

'What do you mean?'

'With respect, I'm afraid I can only speak to Miss Afternoon.'

'That's impossible.'

'That would be regrettable. If I cannot see Miss Afternoon, then I fear I must go instead to the police. As I make it a general rule of life to keep as much distance as possible between myself and the forces of law and order, I should be doubly reluctant to go down that path. Please don't make me.'

Norman scowled.

'What is this bollocks?'

'Oh, well . . .' Philip gave a sad smile. 'At least no one can say I didn't try. I do hope all your licences are in order; I know how distressing a visit from the police can be. Cheerio, Sandy. Good luck, Conchita.'

Philip walked to the exit. His foot was already on the first step when Norman called out to him:

'Hey, wait a sec!'

Philip stopped.

'Yes?'

Norman was staring hard, trying to gauge him. Philip met his gaze levelly, gave nothing away. After a long pause Norman's doubts got the better of him.

'I don't know what this is all about, but . . .' His sharp little eyes flicked over the others in the room. He gave Philip a belated 'Not in front of the children' look. 'Sandy, wake Doris. She'll be in a filthy mood, you'd better take her a coffee.'

'An excellent idea,' said Philip, whose nostrils had already been tickled by the fresh-roasted smell coming from behind the bar. He was hardly able to disguise his elation at Norman's surrender. His information had been spot-on: the consistent breach of all manner of regulations in Bosie Butterflys, Brendan had remarked to him, was so outrageous that it was a wonder the place hadn't been closed down years ago. 'I'll have a coffee, too, please. Caffeine-free, if you've got it, black, no sugar. I'll wait here, shall I?'

'We're working here.'

'I understand,' said Philip, with a glance at Conchita.

'Oh, I don't mind,' said Conchita. 'Nice to have a bit of an audience.'

Norman mumbled something inaudible but almost certainly unfriendly. He turned his back on Philip and sat down at his piano.

'All right, then, let's hear what you've got.'

Philip went to the alcove in the corner, which he had last shared with Seymour. He had an excellent view of the stage. Sandy brought him a coffee, then carried on with the tray towards the curtained entrance behind the piano. Norman pulled him over on the way, and spoke a few words in his ear.

'Can you play "Don't Cry For Me, Argentina"?' Conchita asked, climbing up awkwardly on to the pink stage. 'I've got sheet music, if you need it.'

'Of course I don't bloody need it,' muttered Norman crossly. 'I can play the bloody thing in my sleep, number of times you've come in here and sung it. Let's get a move on!'

He certainly knows how to get the best out of a performer, thought Philip wryly, thinking for a moment of some of his own truly appalling audition experiences. Norman's conspicuous lack of even the slightest redeeming semi-human characteristic should have been enough to secure him instant honorary membership of the Directors' Guild.

Norman began banging the ivories aggressively. He was an accomplished pianist, if unsubtle, but he took the tempo a shade too upbeat and had the singer struggling from the start. Conchita's thin but unobjectionable falsetto began to wobble, and Norman became even more irritated.

'Come on!' he barked as they hit the first chorus. Conchita was thrown completely.

'You're going too fast!'

'Oh, you stupid tart!'

74

Norman jumped up angrily and slammed down the lid of his piano.

'And what if I am too fast – which I'm not – you thick bint! You going to stop in mid-phrase with the club full of punters, go all schoolgirly on me and say, "Could we start again, please?" What's the point of holding open auditions if all we're going to get is rubbish like you? Next time I'll have to put a sign up on the door saying "No Fucking Amateurs". Now pull yourself together, you talentless slag, we'll go from the top again.'

Philip wondered if it was like this at Andrew Lloyd Webber auditions.

'I can't!' Conchita sobbed, wiping his eyes with his sleeve and imprinting in his make-up great tear-stained smudges. He swayed over to the edge of the little stage and slipped down unsteadily to the floor.

'Where you bloody going now?'

'I have to go to the little girls' room . . . to freshen up.'

Conchita kicked off his heels and pattered away to the cloakroom on his rather large bare feet. Norman kicked over his piano stool in disgust.

'These bloody prima donnas!' he muttered in Philip's general direction through clenched teeth. 'Can't take the slightest criticism . . .'

Sandy reappeared through the curtain at the back, bearing the empty tray. He whispered to Norman.

'All right,' said Norman. 'Doris'll see you now.'

Philip took a last sip of his coffee, picked up his Filofax and walked over to the stage. Norman jerked his thumb over his shoulder.

'Top of the stairs. Glass door facing you. And I'll warn you – you'd better have a bloody good reason for getting Doris up at this hour.'

Philip went through the curtain and found himself in a narrow corridor. There were two doors just round the corner to the right, one marked DRESSING ROOM and the other FIRE EXIT. Ahead was a dimly lit staircase, which he took as instructed. Behind him he could hear Norman, calling to the waiting auditionees:

'Melanie Mockingbird! Get your fat arse down here. Fast!'

Philip climbed the stairs. At the first floor, which he surmised was at ground level, there was a door leading off a little landing, but there was no glass in it. He went on up.

The glass door was at the top of the second flight. It was frosted, and almost opaque with dirt. Faded letters spelling out the word 'OFFICE' were just about visible. He knocked on the wooden frame.

'It's open,' said a gruff voice on the other side. Philip went in.

The office was a large but cramped room, overfilled with furniture and filing cabinets, and looking like it hadn't been dusted in years. Behind the half-drawn blinds the windows, which gave out on to a mews, were as grimy as the door. The walls were covered with photographs of Doris Afternoon.

The original was sitting at a once-beautiful mahogany desk, half obscured by mounds of paper. His vast body was shrouded in a voluminous purple kimono. He wore neither wig nor make-up and his face was shockingly white. What little hair he had was shaved to within a millimetre of his scalp.

'Got a light, dear?' he asked, wedging an untipped Camel between his pudgy lips.

'I don't smoke,' said Philip primly, looking for a seat. There was one chair in the corner which bore only a couple of box-files. 'May I?'

Doris nodded and Philip put the boxes on the floor. He pulled up the chair on the other side of the desk and carefully put down his Filofax between two heaps of paper. Meantime, Doris had found a box of matches.

'You'll have to forgive my appearance,' he said, lighting up and inhaling deeply. 'I'm not at my best this time of the morning. I don't usually receive visitors. Norman said it was urgent. Something about Seymour.'

The tone of the voice was crisp and noncommittal. There was none of the archness Philip had heard on Nigel Loseby's tape. And nor was Doris making the slightest effort to flirt. Philip had been keeping his options open as to how to run this scene. He could see no reason not to play it straight.

'I'm here to negotiate for the return of Seymour's diary.'

Doris didn't bat an eyelid.

'The amount of money you're asking is out of the question,' Philip continued, 'but my client is prepared to be reasonable. I am instructed to offer you ten thousand pounds in cash, the money to be delivered today. Considering that the property is not yours to dispose of, the offer is a generous one.'

'Suppose I say I haven't a clue what you're talking about,' said Doris calmly.

Philip didn't answer. He just gave a brittle, sour laugh. Doris stared at him neutrally.

'What exactly is your position in all this, Mr Fletcher?'

'I am merely a disinterested go-between. Nigel Loseby came to me in some distress, as you might imagine. He simply cannot afford to pay the kind of sum you are asking. I can understand how you might assume that he is wealthy, but you are mistaken. He's been in the government for four years. He's ruthlessly ambitious, but he's also squeaky clean, and he lives on his salary. Ten thousand pounds is the most he can afford.'

'Squeaky clean, eh? That's rich! Was coming here your idea or his?'

'Oh, mine alone, and for a very simple reason – Nigel doesn't have the faintest idea who you are. I'm here entirely on my own initiative. Your name has not come

77

up, and nor need it. I can bring you the money, you can give me the diary, and the matter will be sealed and forgotten.'

'That sounds very neat and tidy, Mr Fletcher. Unfortunately it still leaves me with a little problem . . .'

Doris opened a drawer in the desk and took out a bunch of keys. He selected a small one and used it to open a second drawer. After a few moments of rummaging he came out with a handful of small square paper slips. He extended his fist across the desk, and released them in a confetti shower.

'Please, Mr Fletcher, be my guest . . .'

Philip examined one of the slips. It was an IOU for £500 and it bore Seymour's signature. He scanned quickly through the rest of the pile. There were about thirty IOUs in all, some for quite trifling sums, others for rather more. Many were very old, yellowed and dubiously stained. But the signatures were unmistakable.

'They come to twenty-seven thousand and three hundred pounds, give or take the odd shilling,' Doris informed him. 'A significant sum, I'm sure you'll agree. And rather more than the measly ten grand I've just been offered.'

'But still rather less than the hundred and fifty you demanded.'

'Ah, yes. Perhaps I was being a little greedy. You can't really blame me for trying it on, though, can you? But some of these IOUs go back many years. If I were to add up all the interest it perhaps wouldn't sound so unreasonable.'

'Now you really are trying it on . . . What are they for, anyway?'

'Gambling debts.'

'Oh, come on! I knew Seymour for twenty-five years, he never ran up debts like these. We used to play the odd game of poker or pontoon on tour, sometimes we'd even have a flutter on a horse, but he'd never wager more than a few quid. Ever. He wasn't the gambling sort. He didn't have the head for it.'

'You're right, he didn't. It was like the massacre of the innocents, Seymour playing backgammon and roulette. The poor love didn't have a clue.'

'Roulette? Got a gaming licence, have you?'

'Ooh, sharp, aren't we? You don't need a licence at a private party in a private house, Mr Fletcher. You don't think I'd allow anything illegal here at Bosie Butterflys?'

'You count blackmail as legal – do you?'

'Tut-tut!' said Doris with a shake of the head. 'And we were having such a pleasant chat. Why go and spoil it?'

Philip strangled his curt rejoinder at birth. For a moment at the start of the conversation he had had Doris at a disadvantage, but the moment had passed. Doris was in control now, cockiness and campery had by degrees oozed back into the voice. Philip didn't like being teased.

'Mind if I open a window?' he asked with icy politeness as Doris lit another Camel.

'If you must.'

Philip went over to the window, and drew back the blinds enough to get at the catch. He opened it carefully.

'You must know those IOUs have no legal value,' he said matter-of-factly, resuming his seat.

'My lawyer thinks otherwise,' Doris countered. 'He thinks I've a good claim against Seymour's estate. Of which Nigel is the sole beneficiary. I'm just cutting a few corners.'

'And what's your lawyer's opinion on the blackmailing angle?'

'There you go again!'

Doris shook his head sadly. The wounded expression he was putting on failed to convince, if only because he forgot to wipe off his smug look first. Philip felt a strong desire to punch him on the nose.

'Well, what would you call it?' he demanded aggressively. 'If the contents of Seymour's diary come out, it'll ruin Nigel's career, as you know perfectly well – if they were anodyne, they'd have no value. But the figure you're demanding is absurd. It's not worth anything like that and you know it.'

'I've got a provisional offer of a hundred thousand from a Sunday newspaper.'

Philip felt a rush of uncomfortable sensations. It was close in the unventilated dusty room. He felt hot and dry. But across the desk Doris looked cool and unflustered. Was he bluffing? The fat-lidded soft round eyes gave nothing away. How far had he gone already? If he'd spoken to both Nigel and the newspapers, then he couldn't be trusted an inch. And Nigel wasn't going to be able to compete with chequebook journalists. It wasn't fair. Philip was watching his knighthood drift off down the Swanee.

'No paper's going to give you that sort of money,' he said as authoritatively as he was able. 'Not when push comes to shove. They'll talk to their lawyers, and the lawyers will tell them that the diary's not yours to sell. Nigel issues an injunction and their entire print run is jeopardized. It's too great a risk. And if they did run it, and Nigel's career was ruined, then what would he have left to lose? He'd take you to court and sue you for every penny you'd made. Look, I'll level with you: the maximum Nigel can raise, if you give him a week, is twenty thousand pounds. He can still get you half today, as a down payment. That's the absolute ceiling. I'll speak to him about the IOUs. Seymour's estate won't amount to very much, and I think you know that, but I'm sure he could come to some sort of accommodation. It's a damned good offer and it's there on the table. Think about it.'

'All right . . .'

Doris sat back in his chair, the drooping corners of his mouth pursed with amusement. He took a long drag of his cigarette, then crushed it emphatically in the ashtray.

'I've thought about it. No way.'

The verdict was final, with no hope of appeal. Doris might as well have been wearing a black cap.

Philip got up and went to the door. Further conversation would be a waste of breath. He stopped for a moment in the open doorway, his eye on the handle.

'Thank you for your time,' he said politely.

'My pleasure,' came the equally insincere reply. 'I'll give Nigel till the end of next week to match any offer I get from the papers. Till Friday, I can't say any fairer than that now, can I?'

'No, I don't suppose you can.'

Philip closed the glass door behind him and walked down the first flight of stairs. He hesitated at the landing. Down another flight and he'd be back where he'd come from, in the Bosie Butterflys basement. He could hear the unsubtle thump of Norman's piano and the off-key warbling of one of the auditionees. If he went out that way he might have trouble getting in again. But if he wasn't seen to leave now it would arouse suspicion. He went downstairs on tiptoes, opened the door marked FIRE EXIT and saw a staircase beyond that must have led up to street level. He banged it shut as loudly as he could. Then he ran back up to the first-floor landing and went through the other door he'd noticed earlier.

He felt his way along an unlit corridor. There was a locked door on the left, but he spotted the key hanging on a nail nearby. The invitation was irresistible.

He found himself in a garage. A black saloon car filled half of it, the rest was piled high with junk. A small exit, like an airlock, was cut into the heavy folding-door panel. Philip moved a half-full petrol can out of the way, slipped the catch, wedged in a small piece of wood from the floor to prevent it closing behind him, and stepped outside.

He was in the mews he had seen through the office window. It was very small, hardly more than a glorified courtyard. The backs of some offices faced him. The buildings had a run-down, dingy look. He walked out of the mews and stopped on the pavement by the main road. He leant against the nearest of two telephone boxes.

He was desperate for a cigarette. The yearning had started a few minutes earlier, he'd even been tempted to ask Doris for a Camel. It was a shock, after a week of clean living, to feel his nicotine craving burgeoning again. That and the shock of his fruitless interview with Doris had left him feeling quite shaken.

He walked away from the mews, went right and right again, back to the front of the club. There was a newsagents on the corner. He went in and bought himself several packets of sweets. He returned to the mews, resumed his position by the telephones, and stuffed his face with comfort confectionery. A box of fruit pastilles disappeared, and then a tube of wine gums. He was beginning to feel quite sick.

Was Doris bluffing? His instincts told him no. Had Doris thought that *he'd* been bluffing?' His instincts told him yes. Nigel had said that he'd do anything rather than go to court. His career was obviously the only thing he cared about, and if that were ruined even a victory with substantial damages would be no consolation. Had Philip misplayed his hand? Or had he simply underestimated the opposition? Doris was a shrewd customer. He'd know that a sharp lawyer could make any quantity of mud stick in court. And he'd know a few sharp lawyers all right. The law was a lottery. Not only would Nigel's career be finished, he also stood to lose every penny he had.

'Well, that's Plan A up the spout,' Philip reflected aloud, finishing off the last of the wine gums. He checked his watch. He'd been standing there for a good ten minutes now, long enough. It was time to put Plan B into effect.

He walked back into the mews and went in through the garage door. The small wedge of wood was exactly as he had left it. Nor had the inner door been relocked. He locked it now, replacing the key on the nail. He carried on down the corridor, then on out to the landing. He stopped and listened for a moment. The piano playing had stopped. He hurried up the stairs and banged loudly on the office glass door. Without waiting for a reply he went in.

Doris was still behind the desk. Norman was facing him, in the chair Philip had occupied. Both looked at him with predictable astonishment.

'Terribly sorry to trouble you,' said Philip, getting in quickly while they were still off-balance. 'I seem to have left my Filofax behind. Ah yes, I think I can see it – there, on the desk . . .'

He indicated the black leather case, nestled in where he had carefully placed it, between the two heaps of paper. Norman, employing his most natural look, glowered at him suspiciously. Philip just stood by the door, with one hand extended. After a moment Norman picked up the Filofax and brought it over to him.

'Thank you,' said Philip. 'And thank you so much, Norman, for letting me sit in on your auditions earlier. It was most enlightening. Once again, my apologies to you both.'

He clocked the look of distrust on both their faces, smiled blandly and went out and down the stairs, all the way to the bottom. Sandy waved to him from behind the bar, and he waved back. He took the steps up to the main entrance two at a time. No one was left in the lobby. Once outside he headed off rapidly in the direction of Tottenham Court Road. He found a cab at the next corner.

Only in the back of the taxi did he open up the Filofax. The thing itself, the classic yuppie accessory, was an unwanted gift which he would never have dreamt of using. The diary pages themselves were five years out of date. Earlier, at home, he had folded them a few leaves at a time and cut out the centres. The result was crude, but effective enough.

Nigel Loseby's neat little black cassette recorder had fitted almost exactly into the hole. The tape was still turning. Philip put his lips to the microphone and whispered:

'Ha bloody ha!'

7

'He's bluffing, Doris. I knew it was bollocks when he was downstairs demanding to see you.'

'Why'd you let him up then?'

'To be on the safe side. Don't get ratty with me. You handled him, didn't you?'

'Yes, I handled him. He gave me a fright, though.'

'What's Marcus say?'

'Haven't spoken to him yet. Give me a chance!'

'He's not going to like it. Anonymous is one thing. Now young Loseby's rumbled us he'll get rattled.'

'Fletcher claims Loseby knows nothing about it.'

'What do you mean?'

'Says he's acting on his own initiative, like keeping it under his own hat.'

'Bollocks.'

'I'm not so sure. If you ask me, he's trying to put the squeeze on Loseby himself. He knows more than he's letting on.'

'Marcus still isn't going to like it. You know him, he'll start whining about his getting struck off if any of this comes out and do his usual lollipop on a beach act.'

'If any of what I've got on Marcus ever comes out he'll get a sight worse than struck off.'

'Doris, you can't go around blackmailing everyone. You've got to draw the line at your friends.'

'Friends I've got? You must be joking!'

'You've got a point . . . We don't need Marcus, anyway. As long as his journalist friends are kosher.'

'Yes, but they're only going to bite on his say-so, aren't they? Sir Marcus Dalrymple giving them a bell isn't the same as us trying it on now, is it?'

'But what if Loseby gets an injunction, like Fletcher said? They're not going to pay a fistful of dosh for the privilege of sinking themselves up to the neck in shit.'

'He can only get an injunction if he knows which paper it is, can't he? And I'm not going to tell him if you're not. By the time it hits the newsstands it'll be too late.'

'And then Loseby really will have nothing to lose, so at the least we'll be sued for breach of copyright.'

'Which in this case, as Marcus says, is about as murky as murky gets. Look, when all this is out Loseby'll be a broken reed. He's not going to want anyone going over it with a toothcomb in open court, he'll be well out of it. And if what Fletcher told me about his finances is only half true, the poor bugger won't even be able to afford to sue us. Let me tell you this: whatever they might say to the contrary, no tabloid rag is going to mind being sued by a cabinet minister in a case like this. Worst scenario it'll cost them peanuts, but either way the publicity's fantastic. It's a no-lose situation. You know, I think Fletcher might even have done us a favour.'

'Yeah? Well, what's he got to do with any of it, anyway? I don't buy any of this bollocks he's been giving you. What do you say we give Vince a call, get him checked out?'

'My thoughts exactly. He's in the diary, you know.'

'Vince?'

'Of course not! Fletcher, you moron!'

'All right! . . . What'd old Seymour say about him?'

'Quite a lot. He was a catty old queen, was our Seymour. There's a few things about Fletcher sound a bit fishy. Can't quite work it all out.'

'What sort of things?'

'I'll read you a bit. Hang on a sec while I find the right page. There's one near the beginning somewhere. You remember when Richie Calvi copped it?'

'What, that actor?'

'The one who got killed in Bath, at the theatre. The film star. You must remember, there was a real hoo-ha at the time. Seymour was always going on about it.'

'Oh yeah, he was there, wasn't he?'

'He sure was. And so was Fletcher. Listen to this. The entry's a couple of years old. First week in October. Seymour put a big ring round the date, wrote in "Opening Week!" underlined three times next to it. You'll recognize the style. Here we are: "Ricardo mortissimo! Woe, alack, and thrice for effect. Mucho shock horror, headless-chicken-impression contest judges confounded by over-abundance of entrants. Philippo acting dead calm through it all. No wonder rozzers have him down as suspecto numero uno. I know he's acting, but do they? They kept him in nick through half of last night. How long till he cracks? Must try and remember to write to him when he's in Parkhurst. He'll appreciate a pen pal."'

'Nice to have a mate like Seymour, eh? Obviously Fletcher didn't do it, though, or he wouldn't have been trying to bugger us about round here this morning.'

'Your faith in British justice is touching, Norman. They never charged anyone with Calvi's death, you know. Seymour reckoned Fletcher pulled the wool over everyone's eyes. He says they hated each other's guts. There's another long entry, a couple of months later.'

'Doesn't prove anything though, does it?'

'No, but that's not all. Fletcher crops up again at the end. You remember last year, Seymour was working down in Hammersmith? Fletcher was in on that too, and you'll never guess what.'

'Don't tell me there's another dead body!'

'Not quite, but under the usual "Opening Night" underlined three times we get: "Mysterious disappearance in suspicious circumstances. Mel says Phil and Nat dunnit. Mel bonkers, but with Phil around U never can tell."'

'What on earth is all that about?'

'Sounds like gobbledygook, I know, but apparently the director, this Russian bloke, vanished without trace and has never been heard of again. And who were the police most anxious to interview about it? A certain P. Fletcher Esq. Is that coincidence, or have I just got a suspicious nature? There's some more entries, at the end of last year. Really interesting. You see, Seymour had a party – what was that?'

'There's someone at the door.'

'Who the –'

'Terribly sorry to trouble you, I seem to have left my Filofax behind. Ah yes, I think I can see it – there, on the desk . . . Thank you. And thank you so much, Norman, for letting me sit in on your auditions earlier. It was most enlightening. Once again, my apologies to you both . . . . .'

'Ha bloody ha!'

Philip's first reaction was to reach for a drink; his second for a cigarette. With neither to hand he slumped back in his chair and stared lamely out of the window.

The tape had been very faint. At full amplification it had sounded like a scratched old 78 on a wind-up gramophone. It had been enough, though.

Enough, but not enough: why could he have not waited another minute before bursting in to reclaim his wretched Filofax? Then he would have heard the diary entry referring to Seymour's end-of-run party. That had been the night Natasha had told him she was pregnant. Had Seymour guessed the truth? Or had he been eavesdropping, either then or earlier, at the theatre? Seymour had certainly been hanging around outside in the corridor while he and Natasha had been playing a full-blooded scene of passion and recrimination in her dressing room. He had always been one to pop up when you least expected him. And he had fed on gossip like a rose on compost.

Fed on it, then disgorged it with incontinent abandon. Who could tell what he had divulged, or to whom? But that was mere hearsay, green room chatter. Spelt out on paper, embroidered with reasons and deductions, it might prove a different matter, though in a strict legal sense, of course, it would prove nothing at all. That, unfortunately, was not the problem. What if the offending entry ended up in print as part of a Sunday paper's serialization? What if the police found a clue therein to refresh their wilted suspicions? What if, what if, what if? The questions rumbled on in an unending drum-roll.

It was enough to give him a headache. He went to the bathroom and made a selection from his many boxes of aspirin. The broken seals and randomly opened half-used packets bore testimony to a career of hangovers.

'And thus the whirligig of time brings in his revenges . . .'

Philip sat down on the edge of the bath, waiting for his head to clear, watching his face in the mirror above the sink. He had thought he'd been looking fit and spruce this last week, but it had been a delusion. Today he saw only lines.

'To say that all is not going strictly according to plan,' he told himself in a carefully measured Majorish tone, 'would be to understate the case not inconsiderably.'

'Oh yes,' he answered himself with matching dispassion. 'In fact, you've made a right balls-up, haven't you?'

He gave his reflection a painful affirmatory nod. And only a few hours before he'd been thinking just how damned clever he was.

'Why didn't it occur to me that I might feature in the diary? Nigel said his last volume ended three years ago. Since then I've worked twice with Seymour. Two productions, three corpses. A little over the average even for me, and all of it coinciding with the span of that last bloody diary. I can't say I'd have chosen Seymour for my abstract and brief chronicler had I been given the chance. As Nigel has found out, he was never knowingly discreet. I knew that better than anyone. I even used him as a prop in my schemes. I should have been straight round to his flat the day after he died, burned the lot. I'd have missed the big one, though . . .'

And to think it had been there in the room all the while during his interview with Doris; in one of the drawers, perhaps, or lodged amongst the papers on the desk. Had he but caught a glimpse he'd have tucked it under his arm and run off helter-skelter. He could have popped into the stationers and ordered some 'Sir Philip Fletcher' calling cards on the way home.

'Ha bloody ha . . .'

His headache had cleared but he felt nauseous. He needed fresh air. He jumped off the edge of the bath and bolted for the door.

Highbury Fields was deserted. It was a cold day and few of the benches were tenanted, so he was able to pick his spot. He sat where he had sat often before in times past to fulminate and ruminate, but it was hard to think straight. The worm of paranoia was gnawing away inside him.

> Suspicion always haunts the guilty mind;
> The thief doth fear each bush an officer.

The past was another country, and he was by choice an isolationist. The readings from Seymour's diary had raked up in his mind what should have lain undisturbed. He was an actor, a performer, an impersonator; his genius was for the moment, for surfaces and reflections. Seems, madam? Nay, I know not seams . . . He wanted no truck with guilt and fear, those subterranean tunnellers. He could not allow himself to be haunted, not with the queue of ghosts he had waiting in the wings. Softly he murmured the close of Hamlet's soliloquy:

> Thus conscience does make cowards of us all,
> And thus the native hue of resolution
> Is sicklied o'er with the pale cast of thought,
> And enterprises of great pith and moment,
> With this regard their currents turn awry,
> And lose the name of action . . .

The name of action was the only thing he dared not lose. He hadn't got where he was today by passively drifting with the flow. He had not let I dare not wait upon I would, like Lady Macbeth's cat. He had been bloody, bold and resolute. It was the only game in town.

He quit his bench and took off at a brisk pace towards Highbury Grove, banishing the chill from his joints. He passed his old ground-floor flat, but didn't glance inside. There was no room for curiosity or nostalgia on his agenda. He carried on walking, in the direction of Stoke Newington.

The flats he sought were on his left, plain indistinguishable lumps of modern architecture devoid of soul or charm. The first block, Lansbury House, was the one he sought. A group of small children, of mixed race but uniform scruffiness, was clustered on the steps in front of the main entrance.

'Do any of you know George Washington?' Philip asked, with what was for him rare pleasantness: not only did he consider that children, and animals, should be avoided professionally; he was wholeheartedly in favour of extending the principle to his private life as well.

One of the boys, a mop-haired delinquent with a premature boxer's nose, stared at him sullenly. The others all ignored him.

'Let me rephrase that,' said Philip. 'Would any of you like to earn five pounds?'

'Yeah,' answered the sullen kid, springing forward smartly and giving his friends a pre-emptive elbow. 'Me. But if it's drugs I ain't doing nothin' for less than a tenner.'

'Illegal substances are not involved,' responded Philip, who was quietly impressed by the child's grasp of market forces. 'I simply want you to deliver a message. "Ring Philip urgently." Have you got that? Please repeat it.'

'"Ring Philip urgently." Where's the dosh?'

'Don't be impatient. You must be discreet. Do you know George's uncle?'

'The Rev? 'Course I do.'

'It's very important that he doesn't overhear you giving the message to George. Do you understand?'

'Yeah.'

'Good. Here is two pounds fifty. I will give George the rest to give to you when you have passed on the message.'

'No deal. Cash upfront.'

'No. Half upfront, but a one pound bonus if George calls me within the hour.'

'Two.'

'One-fifty. My final offer.'

'Done.'

The boy grabbed the coins from Philip's hand and shot off inside the building. If his nascent criminality failed to bud, Philip reflected, a career as a shop steward beckoned.

Philip returned home and passed the next half-hour in serious contemplation. He weighed his options and evaluated his plans, paying particular attention to emergency procedures. He could be methodical when he wanted to, and he took notes. Those at the top of the page were distilled from an entry he had looked up in his edition of *Who's Who*.

> **Sir Marcus Dalrymple**. Educ. Eton and Christchurch. Solicitor. Senior partner in Dalrymple

Henning & Co. Speciality libel. Author and distin-
guished legal commentator.
Married, one s one d. HOBBIES: Bridge, chess, sailing.
CLUBS: White's, RAC, MCC, Garrick, Bosie
Butterflys.

The last detail, curiously enough, wasn't mentioned in
Who's Who. Dalrymple's full entry, Philip estimated sourly,
was a good three-quarters of an inch longer than his own.
He was actually in the process of measuring it exactly with
a ruler when George rang.

'What you up to then?' George demanded even as he
picked up the receiver.

'I take it you got my message,' Philip answered distractedly. The ruler was confirming his worst suspicions –
the discrepancy might actually be nearer an inch.

'Yeah, I got your message. Wouldn't trust that kid far-
ther'n I could throw him, and the amount of nicked gear
he's usually got in his pockets that ain't far. Why couldn't
you come round yourself, or just give us a bell?'

'I'm not exactly popular in your household, George. If
your uncle picked up the phone I'd only have to hang up,
and that would look suspicious now, wouldn't it?'

'My uncle says you are Lucifer's chosen representative
in the Highbury and Islington area.'

'How kind of him,' said Philip, a little taken aback. Dev-
ilry by postal code was a new concept to him. The Rev.
Cornelius Washington was clearly a man of an original cast
of mind, and the least excuse he gave him to exercise it
the better. The wisdom of his furtive method of contact
was confirmed.

'George, I need you to do a job for me. Tonight. I trust
you're free.'

'What sort of job?'

'You know perfectly well.'

George hesitated.

'I ain't done nothing dodgy in a long time, you know that.'

'On the contrary, you did it last week.'

'What you talking about?'

'I'm talking about you breaking into my flat.'

'That's different!'

'Qualitatively perhaps, but not quantitatively.'

'You what?'

'You may be rusty, but you haven't lost the knack. It's very urgent, George, and I'll be very grateful.'

George hesitated again, but not very convincingly.

'How grateful?'

'Five hundred pounds. An end to your financial problems. As described in your letter.'

This time the hesitation was fractional.

'All right . . . You want me to nick a motor?'

'Certainly not!'

'No extra charge.'

'After last time? You must be joking. We'll take a cab. Meet me at Highbury Corner at half past two tomorrow morning.'

'Half past two! You joking!'

'George, criminality isn't a nine-to-five occupation, as you know full well. Bring all the usual equipment. I don't expect any complications. I owe that kid who passed on my message four pounds. Will you give it to him and I'll pay you back.'

'Four quid? You were done, mate! See you later!'

George was still laughing as Philip put down the receiver on him. He turned his ruler round and remeasured Sir Marcus Dalrymple's entry in centimetres just to be sure. Then he checked his own meagre paragraph one last time.

It would look a very great deal better, he reflected, under the rather grander heading 'Sir Philip Fletcher'.

8

Philip paid off the cab at Euston and they walked from there. The night was dry, but cold, and the streets past Tottenham Court Road empty. They went at a brisk pace, in silence, and reached the club just after 3.00 a.m. Philip left George in a doorway at the front while he went round to the mews to reconnoitre.

Only the faintest bleeding from the streetlamps seeped into the courtyard. The buildings appeared as monolithic black slabs; no lights behind the windows. The club stayed open till 2.00 a.m. at weekends; till 12.00 p.m. during the week. When Philip was sure that he could detect no signs of life he went to the street corner and beckoned George to join him.

They felt their way along the wall and stopped outside the garage door. Philip whispered in George's ear.

'It's the room directly above. Standard catches on the windows, Yale on the door. I'd rather you didn't smash the glass.'

'That's for amateurs. What about alarms?'

'There's a contact pad in the garage door. Light detector on the lower landing going down into the club – you don't have to go anywhere near it. Nothing else that I saw. I checked it pretty thoroughly this morning.'

'Sounds like it. Right. I'll get in up there, come down and open the garage for you.'

'What about the contact pad?'

'Don't worry about it. Is it at the top or the bottom of the door?'

'Bottom. About three inches up. The key into the garage is in the corridor next to the door, on a nail.'

'Sounds like a piece of piss, mate. Give us a leg up, will you?'

Philip put his back to the wall and cupped his hands while George stuck in a foot.

'Ouch!' said Philip, as George climbed up on to his shoulders, using his head for leverage. The boy weighed far more than his skinny frame suggested.

'Ssh!' he hissed back, while Philip blinked the tears from his eyes. 'It's only for a sec.'

He was as good as his word. The weight was lifted suddenly from Philip's shoulders as George appeared somehow to slither up the wall. Philip supposed that he must have spotted some sort of ledge to cling to. He could vaguely sense the shape of the body hovering above him, and just as vaguely hear the delicate scratching of metal on metal.

Perhaps five minutes passed. In the total darkness it felt like much longer. Philip spent the time doing simple breathing exercises, trying to keep himself calm.

He heard the bolts being drawn on the inside of the garage door, and then it opened, slowly. A pencil flashlight was pointing out, the beam aimed downwards at the base of the door frame, where George was crouching.

'Get in then!' he whispered urgently. 'Can't hold on to this all night!'

Philip did as he was told, and then closed the door, carefully, again under instruction. By the flashlight he saw that George was holding a thin metal strip, the base covered with coiled wire, against the alarm pad. He withdrew it carefully once the door was closed and the proper contact re-established.

'Easy when you know how,' he confided nonchalantly.

'Takes a bit of practice though – magnetic, you see, one slip and you bugger up your north-south polarities. You know where you're going, I take it?'

Philip led the way back up to the first floor, where George had already infiltrated the Yale lock. They went into the office.

'Keep a lookout, will you?' he said, taking his own torch from his pocket. 'I'll try and be quick.'

He would try, but it wasn't going to be easy: since the morning, the junk on Doris's desk seemed to have bred and multiplied. Files, papers, books; all were strewn about in random and precariously balanced piles. One false touch and the lot would come tumbling down. Philip approached the task like a dentist engaged in a delicate extraction.

He found nothing. A large manila envelope got his pulse up for a moment, but the flash of red inside turned out to be a cardboard divider. He replaced the envelope where he had found it, wedged between two leaning towers of paper, and focused his attention on the drawers.

The one on the top left was open and contained the keys to the others. The main centre drawer held Seymour's IOU slips, and a diary – but not the one he sought. He glanced through it anyway, and a couple of entries caught his eye. He turned his attention to the drawer on the right, the deepest, which was revealed as a drinks cabinet. His torch lingered fondly on the near-full bottle of malt whisky. He closed the door reluctantly.

'Nothing,' he whispered to George, joining him at the door. 'I'm afraid I'm going to have to look around some more.'

'I ain't got nothing better to do,' came the casual reply.

Philip turned his attention to the bookshelves behind the desk, in which books were noticeably thin on the ground. The paper mounds yielded nothing but dust. His dry tongue pined for the Scotch in the drawer.

What had he expected? It had been naive of him to

suppose that because the diary had been there earlier it would be there tonight. His visit would have put Doris and Norman on guard. He should have burgled the place yesterday, saved the face-to-face confrontation till later. But then he wouldn't have been able to check out the alarm system. No, the strategy had been correct, he'd cocked up with the tactics. He had to admit that thus far in l'affaire Loseby his performance had been well under par.

Only a small metal filing cabinet in the corner remained. He approached it leadenly, almost afraid to confirm its emptiness. It was locked.

'George . . .'

The simple lock was child's play to someone of George's accomplishments. He inserted what looked like the filed-down tip of a coathanger into the hole and jiggled it open. The drawer was empty.

'Try the others, please.'

They were all empty. Philip sighed and sat back against the wall. He wondered if he could be bothered to poke around under the carpets.

'That's odd,' George murmured, rattling the filing cabinet gently.

'How do you mean?'

'Well, look at this place. Junk everywhere, all the drawers in that desk you were looking in bursting with it. What's this doing here empty?'

'Maybe they just bought it.'

'No, it's old. Here, hold this.'

Philip took his flashlight while George pulled the cabinet over to one side and walked it away from the wall. He shone both torches into the space behind.

'Well done,' he murmured appreciatively.

A wall safe was revealed, a black lustreless metal door fronted by an upright steel handle. George took back his torch and examined it carefully.

'Ain't much I can do with this, I'm afraid. You'd need a jelly man to get in there.'

Philip shone his own torch at the lock.

'It's not like you, George. If it were a combination I could understand, but this looks common or garden to me.'

'No, you're wrong. I could bugger around all night with this and not get anywhere. Even a pro safecracker would have to blow it, and I'm not in that league. Only other way in is with the key. Unless they left it lying in one of them drawers, I can't help. It'd be a big, heavy, solid bastard – you couldn't miss it.'

There hadn't been anything that fitted George's description in the desk; only the little bunch of desk keys. It was hardly likely they'd have been left around, in any case, not if there was anything valuable in the safe. And an almost overwhelming psychic intuition told Philip that there was.

'Damn, it looks like it'll have to be Plan C . . .'

'You what?'

The only drawback was that he didn't actually have a Plan C. Arson, perhaps? No, they'd probably fish the safe out of the wreckage, toasted but unharmed. Or someone could get killed, prompting a murder investigation and raising the stakes so high that Nigel Loseby might crack. The ramifications were endless; none of the possibilities appealed. He was getting himself into ever murkier waters, swimming further out of his depth with every stroke. A rare and unwelcome feeling of hopelessness engulfed him.

A light came on out in the corridor. George's frozen form became suddenly visible against the glass door panel. Philip had to give him a nudge. They both turned off their torches together.

The corridor outside was carpeted, they didn't hear any footsteps. But a floorboard creaked, and then another, nearer. A shape appeared in the door panel.

It seemed to hang there, unmoving, like a forgotten character in a shadow play. Then it gave a deep hoarse cough, at which the glass trembled. And then it moved on.

A door was banged further down the corridor. A minute passed. Philip sat back on his aching haunches, hardly breathing, his eyes fixed on George's motionless outline. The sound of a toilet flushing rumbled through the wall.

The door down the corridor was opened again, emitting a rush of noise from the cistern. The shadow of Doris – the bulk permitted no doubt as to ownership – billowed across the door heading back whence it had come, and a few moments later the light in the corridor was extinguished.

They both sat in silence, listening to each other's breathing. At length, and simultaneously, they both let out a long sigh.

'I think we'll leave now,' said Philip wisely.

'You don't want to go in and heavy him up, get the key that way?'

'No, I do not . . .'

Physical violence was hardly his forte, and nor, despite the bravado, did he think it was George's. He suspected that Doris could have probably disabled them both with one meaty forearm smash. Whatever Plan C might turn out to be, it wouldn't include a fortnight in plaster.

They gave it a few more minutes, and then they slipped out of the door, Philip declining George's suggestion that he might like to follow him out of the window and down the drainpipe. He reckoned that he had compromised his dignity quite enough for one night already.

They didn't dare use their flashlights, but crept along to the top of the staircase in darkness. They went on tiptoe, wary of the noisy floorboards. They could feel each other's tension.

'What was that?' George gasped suddenly, grabbing Philip's arm and squeezing it very hard.

The mixture of shock and pain almost made Philip yelp. He threw off George's grip crossly.

'How should I know?' he hissed back. 'Quiet!'

They heard the noise again: muffled but distressed, like an animal whimper. It came from the other end of the corridor.

'I'm getting out of here,' whispered George frantically. 'This place gives me the spooks.'

'You go on ahead,' Philip murmured back. 'I'll join you down in the garage – if you'll be so good as to wait for me.'

'What? What you up to?'

'Keep your voice down, or we'll be heard! I just want to do a little more reconnaissance, that's all. Don't argue, just go on down.'

George left reluctantly, muttering under his breath. Philip ignored him. The night's work had cost him £500, thus far for nothing; he might as well at least try and get some return on his investment.

Philip proceeded down the corridor. He heard the whimpering noise repeated, at irregular intervals, gradually getting closer. The faintest glimmer of light must have been coming from somewhere, because at the end of the corridor he could just make out the shape of the wall. There was a right-angled turn. He peeped around it cautiously.

Ahead of him lay another stretch of landing, uncarpeted, at the end of which was a solid white door. It stood an inch or so ajar, with light flooding out of the gap. It was the source of the noise they'd heard.

And of other noises too: a faint rhythmic swishing sound, and an occasional indistinct voice, also muffled. Philip approached carefully, conscious that if anyone came out now he'd have no warning and the night's work would be blown, but too intrigued to hold himself back. He became aware of movement on the other side of the door. He held his breath and put his eye to the crack.

Swish! went the noise of Doris's riding crop. Thwack! came the answer from Norman's skinny bare buttocks.

'Naughty boy!' said Doris. 'You've been a very, very naughty boy!'

101

That the voice was indistinct was hardly surprising, given that its owner was wearing a full-face rubber diving mask. The features were equally blurred behind the misted glass.

'Naughty! Naughty! Naughty!'

Swish! Thwack! Argh!

The groans came from Norman, who was lying naked and spreadeagled on the bed, his wrists and ankles bound to the four corners and a thick band of brown sticky tape stuck over his mouth. Doris was kneeling across his back to administer punishment, a hideous parody of perversion in rubber corsetry and silk stockings. Philip was irresistibly reminded of Hieronymus Bosch.

'All places shall be hell that are not heaven,' he whispered to himself, though he'd have been quite safe to speak aloud: Doris and Norman probably wouldn't have noticed an earthquake.

'There's only one thing to do with naughty boys like you!' mumbled Doris sternly, lifting his fat knees from Norman's spine and struggling to get his feet up on to the bed. He managed this with considerable difficulty, and not merely on account of his unwieldy bulk: a pair of rubber flippers was attached to his feet. The diving look was obviously in this year.

'You leave me no option!' declared Doris with petulant regret. 'This is going to hurt you a great deal more than it's going to hurt me, I'm pleased to say.'

He bent down with extreme awkwardness and took off one of the rubber flippers. Norman's eyes bulged in anticipation and he started whooping into his gag like a chimpanzee. But Doris was not inclined to show mercy.

'Take that, you little swine! And that!'

Doris had dropped his riding crop and was spanking Norman's bottom viciously with the flipper. Philip, who had never been shocked by anything to do with sex in his life, was nonetheless extremely surprised.

He turned away and retraced his steps down the corridor,

no longer worrying overmuch about the squeaking floorboards. He felt his way down the stairs and along to the garage. George was just inside the door, leaning against the bonnet of the black saloon.

'See what you wanted to?' he asked, sounding somewhat peeved.

'Not exactly,' Philip answered. 'Shall we go?'

George negotiated his way through the alarm system one last time and they stepped out into the mews. Philip stood quietly for a moment, taking in the fresh night air. He felt like he needed it.

They walked back towards Euston, where they picked up a cab. Philip sat in silence all the way back, thinking. He dropped George off, then took the taxi on home. It was gone 4.30 by the time he got in.

But he didn't sleep. Instead he sat at his desk, where his copy of *Who's Who* lay open, the place marked by his tape measure. He pushed it to one side and examined his notes. He picked up his pencil, and wrote at the top of a blank sheet in block capitals:

PLAN C

Some time later, as the dull light of dawn was beginning to show through the curtains, an idea as desperate as any he had conceived in his long years of sub-legal scheming had begun to take shape in the devious recesses of his brain.

9

Three drag queens, a blonde, a redhead and a brunette, were sitting in the foyer of Bosie Butterflys. The distant sound of a piano came tinkling up the stairs from beneath, punctuated by Norman's aggressive outbursts of nasal whine.

'Gives me the willies just hearing his voice,' whispered the redhead with a shiver. 'It's more than I can bear to face him first thing in the morning.'

'I expect it's better than facing him last thing at night, dear,' answered the brunette archly. 'Imagine nodding off with that on the pillow next to you.'

'Don't! You'll give me nightmares!'

They both laughed nervously. Each angled a sidelong look at the blonde, who sat impassively and a little apart. The two exchanged knowing glances.

'Do you know the score here then, love?' asked the brunette, sympathetically.

The blonde head turned to take them in with a slow imperious sweep. The chin was tilted haughtily, the eyes glacial and uncompromising. A superciliously raised eyebrow seemed to imply surprise at being thus addressed. An awkward pause ensued.

'Sorry, it's just that we haven't seen you around,' murmured the brunette uncomfortably. 'We all know each other, you see, and well . . . sorry, we ought to have intro-duced ourselves properly: I'm Melanie Mockingbird.'

'And I'm Rita Hepburn,' said the redhead.

After another momentary pause the ghost of a smile flitted across the blonde's exquisitely glossed lips.

'Und I am Marlene von Trapp,' said Philip Fletcher in a brittle Teutonic tone.

The forced nature of the smile was not exclusively due to social *froideur*: Philip's bra strap was killing him.

'Ooh, that's nice,' said Rita kindly. 'Nice name, don't you think?'

'Very nice,' agreed Melanie. 'So where you from, Marlene?'

'Heidelberg.'

'That's nice. What sort of act do you do?'

'High. Class.' Philip answered, punctuating his answer emphatically. His tone and look suggested that only a brave soul would have dared suggest otherwise. Rita and Melanie were not cut from an heroic cloth.

'Oh, of course, yes,' said Rita hastily. 'That goes without saying. You, er, you've not been down here before though, have you?'

'Nein.'

'I think we'd better warn you: that Norman, downstairs, he's a real little Hitler . . . oops, I'm sorry! I didn't mean to say that!'

Rita's complexion had come out in sympathy with his wig; Melanie looked merely ashen.

'Don't mind my friend,' he said, cravenly shifting his seat to put a little distance between them. 'The point is that with old Norm his bark is worse than his bite. You shouldn't let him upset you, that's all.'

'I von't,' responded Philip coolly. 'Do zey usually keep you hanging around zis long?'

'Ooh, I know, they're awful!' said Rita, with feeling. 'I've wasted hours in here before! Have you got somewhere to go on to?'

'No. It's just zat I left my panzer on a meter.'

Melanie gave a nervous titter. Rita looked as if he didn't know whether to laugh or cry. There was an awkward pause.

'Been to London before?' asked Melanie, gamely trying to keep the conversation rolling.

'Nein. But my father has visited often.'

'On pleasure or business?'

'Business. He flew with the Luftwaffe.'

'Ah . . .'

Philip hoped that as conversation killers went, this one might prove terminal. But Melanie was persistent.

'Got somewhere nice to stay?' he asked after only a token silence.

'Hotel,' Philip answered carefully. 'In Bayswater.'

'Ooh, bit expensive, that! You'll be wanting to move, I expect. That is, if you're going to be here long. We know a place, if you're interested, don't we, Rita?'

'Oh, yes . . .' offered Rita, without evident enthusiasm.

Philip hesitated. As it happened the hotel was quite cheap, but it was poky and insalubrious. He'd also received some none too friendly looks when he'd gone out an hour ago cross-dressed to the nines.

'It's not very grand,' explained Melanie, 'but it's friendly.'

'Vere is zis place, please?'

'Cumberland Mansions. Just behind Marylebone Station. We both live there.'

'I need my own space, you understand?'

'Oh yes, I'm not asking you to share or anything. It's a self-contained flat, belongs to a friend of ours, called Conchita. She's gone to Brazil, for a couple of months. It came up very suddenly. You know . . .'

'I know vat?'

'You know, Brazil. Where the nuts are.'

Rita gave another of his girlish giggles. Melanie leant towards Philip and whispered softly:

'She's gone for the operation.'

'Ah yes. Of course.'

The nature of the operation did not need to be specified. It wasn't the kind of thing one could get on the National Health.

'It'd only be temporary, of course, till Conchita comes back, but because it's such a short let she couldn't do a thing with it. It's small but clean – very discreet neighbours. I'm sure you'd love it.'

'Tanks. Perhaps it depends on how I get along here, you understand? In any case, I vill think about it.'

'Oh do! I'll give you my number, I think I've got a card on me. Yes, here.'

Melanie took a card out of his handbag and passed it over. Philip put it into his own handbag. He'd never appreciated just how useful they were until now.

Norman's sweet tones came wafting up the stairs:

'Marlene von Trapp! Get down here! Fast!'

'At last!' muttered Philip emphatically, rising in his own time and proceeding to the top of the stairs.

'Good luck,' said Rita dutifully.

'Tanks. I shouldn't think I'll need it.'

Philip turned with a disdainful toss of the head and left Rita wilting into the carpet. He began the long slow descent of the stairs.

Like Conchita, whom he had accompanied on the same journey only two days ago, he went down in a kind of awkward sideways shuffle, distrustful of his ability to balance on heels. His ankle-length gown so confined his thighs that he felt as if he were bandaged. He clung tightly to the banister for support.

'I'm going to a fancy-dress party,' Philip had lied to his old friend Denis, first thing Monday morning. 'It's not really me, I know, but I need something in the gender-bending line.'

'You mean a tarts and vicars job?' asked his old dresser sagely.

'A little more upmarket than that. Could you manage a screen goddess?'

'With your legs, love? You'll be lucky!'

Philip had presumed Denis was joking. His regime of exercise and healthy living had delivered him into a state of near physical perfection.

'Have you decided on your colouring?' Denis asked him. Philip shook his head. 'I think you should be blonde. Blondes have more fun, the lucky things! Got a wig?'

'Not yet.'

'Then I'll send you down to see Algy later. But first, let's get you a frock . . .'

Fortunately the theatrical costumiers where Denis now worked was full of frocks. Even accounting for Philip's unfeminine measurements, the choice, allowing for a touch of nipping and tucking, was encyclopaedic. After much soul- and rail-searching Denis had alighted on a cobalt-blue thirties evening gown that shimmered like fish-scales on the hanger.

'Could have been made for you,' Denis opined when Philip had tried it on. 'Get that blonde rug on and we'll have every Marilyn wannabe in London scratching your eyes out!'

It wasn't one of Philip's dearest ambitions. When Algy offered him Marlene rather than Marilyn he was happy to accede.

'Yes, I think it's more you, really, the statuesque look,' said Algy thoughtfully, brushing through the long platinum locks. 'Ooh, look at those hands. We've got to do something about them!'

And so Philip had been sent to Lenny for a manicure, and afterwards to Arthur for some shoes, and last of all to Lavinia, in corsetry, who, though a genuine woman in her natural right, had breathed the camp air around her for so many years that her effeminacy seemed more oddly artificial than anyone else's. All theatrical costumiers are like this; it's not even optional.

And so Philip Fletcher, in Algy's wig and Arthur's shoes and Denis's frock, emerged unsteadily into the basement of Bosie Butterflys, a club of which they had all heard but which (as he had learnt through delicate probing after bringing up the subject of Seymour's demise) they never frequented. He paused for a moment on the bottom step to compose himself.

'Bloody hell!' exclaimed Norman from the other end of the room. 'What we got here? Brünnhilde the bleeding Valkyrie?'

'Und who are you zen?' drawled back Philip. 'Ze dwarf of ze Nibelungen in person?'

Philip felt the sudden quiet in the stale air: at the bar Sandy paused in the act of placing a just-dried glass on a tray; behind him a second barman stood frozen with both arms plunged to the elbow in the washing-up. Norman himself sat at his piano stool, with his jaw dropping down to the keys. Idly draping his chiffon scarf over his shoulder, Philip sauntered across to him; or at least gave as good an impression of a saunter as he was able to manage on three-inch heels.

'You actually play zat honky tonk, liebling, or iss it just for show?'

Norman's face, which had been transfixed into stillness, began suddenly to twitch at the corners. The pupils dilated furiously.

'This someone's idea of a wind-up? One of you lot behind the bar getting this on video, or what?'

'Viz a face like yours, munchkin? You'll be lucky!'

With a haughty flick of his wig Philip turned away and mounted the steps at the front of the pink stage. He stopped in front of the microphone and adjusted the height of the stand. Out of the corner of his eye he saw Norman rising from his piano stool.

'Sorry, am I missing something here?' he demanded with overstressed incredulity, rolling his eyes and opening his palms to the room in general. 'Who's in charge of these auditions, you or me?'

'Since you ask . . .' said Philip crisply, holding the microphone up in his left hand and gathering the flex in his right. 'I am!'

He jerked his arm suddenly, snapping the flex across the floor. It cracked like a whip.

'Sit!' he commanded sternly. 'Und play!'

Norman looked as if he wanted to protest, but it was already too late: whether it had been the smack in the flex or the smack in the voice it was hard to say, but whichever, he had sat back down with instinctive obedience at his piano. He looked baffled, like an old dog who had unconsciously performed a new trick; and Philip had no intention of loosening his leash.

'I vill give you "Moon of Alabama" by Brecht und Weill, ja? On ze count of three, now, und don't keep me hanging about if you know vat's gut for you – ein, zwei, drei!'

Philip flicked his flex again for good measure. Norman began to play.

'Too slow! Schnell! Schnell! Take it again, from ze top – ein, zwei, drei!'

Crack went the flex and Norman began to thump the ivories with gusto. Philip belted out the song at a pace that would have had Lotte Lenya gasping for breath, even in the slow passage.

Faster, of course, didn't necessarily mean better, but Philip hoped that speed might detract at least a little from the rough edges in his voice.

He wasn't a natural born singer, but he could put a song over, like any decent actor, given a little coaching and rehearsal. He had spent all of Sunday and Monday afternoons with a pianist friend who was currently musical director of a West End show. It may not have turned him from an ugly duckling into a swan, but it had smoothed his feathers.

He hit the last few lines aggressively. It was a music best served raw, which at least suited his limited vocal skills. As Norman's final chords floated away, a smattering of applause sounded from behind the bar. Philip inclined his head with a Prussian nod to Sandy and friend.

'Vell?' he demanded of Norman.

Norman hesitated. He was still looking shell-shocked.

'What else do you do?' he asked sheepishly.

'Vat else do you vant?'

'Er, Lili Marleen?'

'Ha! Zat old tear-jerker. You vant it in English or German?'

'What's best?'

'German, you dummkopf! German iss best for cabaret.'

'You can do all that decadent stuff, then?'

'Decadent, darlink, iss my middle name . . .'

Philip stepped down from the stage with as languid an air of decadence as a man in a dress might reasonably be expected to muster at eleven o'clock of a Tuesday morning.

'Ven vould you like me to start?'

'Well . . .' Norman consulted a sheaf of papers on top of the piano. 'I think we've got a vacancy Friday –'

'I am not in London forever, you know!' declared Philip shrilly, hands on hips.

'Oh right, well . . . I daresay we could fit you in then. What about tomorrow? Just for a short set, a couple of numbers only, but that's the way we always do things here, with a new act, break it in gradually, it's nothing –'

'Zat iss fine,' said Philip, breathing an inward sigh of relief: at least he'd have time to learn Lili Marleen, either in English or German. 'I vill see you tomorrow. At vat time?'

'Can you get here for five o'clock for a quick rehearsal. I'll let you know then where we can slot you in.'

'Gut. Till tomorrow.'

'Er, Marlene!'

Philip stopped on his way to the staircase. He glanced pointedly at his watch, an elegant ladies' Cartier that had been resident in his bedside table drawer since its owner had forgotten to reattach it to her wrist after a night of fondly remembered debauchery.

'You can go out the other way if you like,' Norman mumbled, indicating the door behind the piano. 'That's the artistes' entrance.'

'I vill go zis vay. I haf left my coat.'

'Oh right – and Marlene!'

Philip stopped again. He tapped his feet impatiently.

'Ja?'

'We need a phone number. In case we have to contact you.'

'I vill give you a number tomorrow. Consider yourself lucky – I don't give it to every man I meet. Auf wiedersehen!'

He exited grandly up the stairs, leaving in his wake a cloud of disdain mixed with the Chanel No. 5 another lady friend had left in his bathroom cabinet.

'How'd you get on then?' asked Melanie eagerly as he reached the top of the stairs. Philip shrugged.

'Not so bad. Now let us talk for a minute before I go: about zat flat . . .'

10

The flat was on the fourth floor, one below the top. It contained two small rooms, a bathroom of equal size and disproportionate luxuriousness, and a miniature kitchen. The narrow windows admitted a little light into the living room, almost none at all into the bedroom, where the subdued lilac wallpaper emanated a morbid air.

'It's far from grand, I know,' apologized Melanie for the umpteenth time, 'but it's homely.'

Funeral homely, Philip surmised. It was neat, it was clean, and it was quiet, although the much larger flat which Melanie shared with Rita was only two floors down, and keeping his distance might prove difficult. Melanie seemed so indifferent to the casual unfriendliness of his manner that he was beginning to feel guilty.

'How much?' he demanded with strangled curtness. He was prepared to haggle.

'Forty pounds a week. That's without heating – there's a gas meter.'

With or without gas it wasn't worth arguing about. Melanie explained that they all enjoyed protected tenancies.

'We've been here for yonks, you see. Landlords were going to tear the place down, redevelop it for yuppies, but they ran out of money, thank God! Don't know where we'd find anywhere this convenient again.'

'Convenient for Bosie Butterflys?'

'Well, I just mean central, you know . . . I don't get a lot at Bosie's, to be honest, nor did Conchita. It's a very popular club, they only take top acts. You must be brilliant to have got in there at the first attempt.'

'Tanks,' said Philip, who was never averse to praise, whatever the circumstances.

'So what do you think?' asked Melanie, indicating the flat with a wave of his thick, ringed fingers.

'Sehr gut,' answered Philip with a nod. 'I vill take it. You vant cash in advance?'

Just a week's rent would do, Melanie informed him kindly. After all, they were sisters under the skin. Philip took £40 from his purse.

'So you work the German circuit usually, do you?' Melanie asked, putting the money away in his bag. He looked as if he might be about to park his ample bottom on the floral-covered armchair by the door. He certainly didn't look as if he had the slightest intention of leaving. Philip pretended to notice his watch:

'Ach! Is zat ze time?'

'Oh, I'm terribly sorry, am I intruding? If you'd like me to leave – '

'Yes, please!'

Philip stepped smartly to the door, and held it open. Melanie exited wearing an expression of disappointment.

'If there's anything you want, anything at all – '

'I vill call,' replied Philip firmly, and closed the door.

He was sure that Melanie would prove useful to him as a source of information, but right now he didn't have time to chat. The glance at the watch had not been entirely faked. He still had a busy day ahead of him.

He took his one suitcase into the bedroom and unpacked it, which didn't take long. Besides the blue evening dress and high-heeled shoes it contained only make-up, a wash-bag and underwear, male and female. He was wearing the rest of his wardrobe, a plain black jacket with matching knee-length skirt, a white blouse and comfortable court shoes. He would need to buy some stockings urgently; the pair he had on was already laddering.

He sat down at Conchita's dressing table to see to his make-up. It was a little heavy, he decided, over-rouged and over-mascara'd. He wiped off the bright red lipstick and tried one of the subtler shades Lavinia had recommended. He looked better already. He touched up his nails and his eyes.

He didn't recognize himself in the mirror. The way the long wig framed his features made even the shape of his face seem different. The accent of his make-up distorted his lips, cheeks, eyes; only the line of the nose seemed at all familiar. He was used to disguising himself, he had proved himself a master of concealment both on and off the stage, but this transformation was more extreme than any he had previously attempted. He sensed no point of contact with the hybrid reflection now glancing back at him. Because he felt so uninvolved, he hoped it would be easier to carry it off, to disguise his deep inner trepidation.

He put on the long camel coat Denis had given him, a shapeless black bonnet that covered his ears, and a pair of dark glasses. Suitably layered against the outside world, he left his new flat for the first time.

He went down by the stairs, partly to avoid the possibility of being in the lift with a stranger (or Melanie for that matter); partly just to get his bearings. The corridors were dark and thinly carpeted; the plain closed doors gave no clue as to who or what might lie beyond them. The block, a warren of hermetically sealed units, seemed to be as discreet as advertised.

He stepped out of the dark communal entrance into the street, automatically pulling his wide lapel up to his chin. The day was blustery, but it was a gesture of psychological, not material, defence. He had not yet found his feet with this performance.

115

His anxieties bubbled up as soon as he hailed a taxi. As the cab slowed and he caught the driver's eye, he felt suddenly uncovered. The casual appraising look, such as he had given countless times to women strangers, turned in a flash from moderate interest to cold disdain. Philip sensed that he was tempted just to drive off and refuse the fare. The second he closed the door behind him the cab moved off abruptly, throwing him off-balance into the seat. The driver raised a hand and casually flipped the glass partition shut. Philip felt humiliated.

He paid off the cab at Highbury Corner and walked across the Fields, a bundle of paranoid nerves. He was convinced that every eye was boring through him, everyone he passed was filled with instant distaste. It was one thing to sustain the performance in the artificial closed environment of Bosie Butterflys, but the real world was unforgiving. He barely checked that the coast was clear, but bolted straight up to his flat. Fortunately he passed no one on the stair, no inquisitive neighbour who might guess the sordid secret of Philip Fletcher.

It was a relief to remove the wig; the gauze was soaked with sweat. He tore off his skirt and blouse, ran to the bathroom and applied cream to his face, wiping away his cosmetic covering. He started to run a bath, then went to check his machine.

There was a message from George, saying he'd been round earlier to say goodbye, he was going back to Manchester on the evening train and he was sorry to have missed him. Philip supposed he should have been thankful that George hadn't been in the flat. The boy seemed to break in with such casual regularity it would have been just his luck to have been caught in full transvestite rig. Somehow he didn't think that George would have believed his explanations.

There was also a terse message from Nigel Loseby. Philip rang the House of Commons and spoke to his secretary.

He was in the bathroom, nursing the water to its optimum temperature, when the junior minister rang him back.

'That was quick,' Philip commented, taking the call from his bedroom.

'I don't have much time,' came the brusque reply. 'I'm meant to be in a meeting. What have you found out?'

'Not a lot, I'm afraid,' answered Philip carefully. 'Had any more phone calls?'

'Oh yes,' came the bitter answer. 'I've been screening them, as you advised, but one slipped through my secretary's net this morning. He claimed to be my new constituency chairman.'

'Cunning,' opined Philip, who was willing to give credit where it was due.

'Gave me a hell of a shock, I'll tell you. They'd obviously done their research. It was a different voice this time. There must be a gang.'

'What sort of a voice?'

'Hard to describe. Unpleasant, I can say that much. The kind of voice a rat would have if it could talk.'

Philip thought he recognized an accurate description of Norman's exquisite tones.

'What did he say?'

'He said I might not enjoy what I was going to read in one of the Sunday tabloids. He said that they were still willing to give me a chance to match the offer and that I had until Friday. I told him he could expect to see me in court. He suggested that if I were having trouble raising the money I might be in even more trouble trying to pay my legal fees, though he did kindly point out that that was really a secondary issue. He wished me luck in searching for a new job. Very thoughtful of him. Just who the hell are these people?'

Philip was relieved. Norman might have blown his gaff, taunted Nigel with his choice of emissary. If he'd let on to Nigel that Philip had been to see them, it would have put him in a very poor light indeed. He supposed that Norman had been checking out the story he'd told Doris as well as keeping tabs on Nigel.

'I'm following up some leads,' said Philip, attempting to sound soothing. 'If they call again, just stall them – and don't panic.'

It was easier advice to give than to receive. Nigel sounded dubious and depressed. Philip listened patiently to his mournful ramblings for a minute more and then he had to go back to his meeting.

Philip stood cradling the telephone, thinking. Was there any mileage in playing both ends against the middle? Wouldn't it have been easier, and safer, to come clean with Nigel and tell him all he knew? Safer, but not in his nature. Secrecy and furtiveness were among his basic instincts: he was a conjuror by temperament; something of a juggler, too. He would keep all his balls in the air just in case, like a qualified Micawber; something might turn up. But if it did, he hoped it would be sooner rather than later. He wasn't sure how much to believe Norman's boast about the Sunday tabloid, but he would have to act as if expecting the worst. Today was Tuesday. That left him only three days. It wasn't a cheering prospect.

He had just put down the phone and was on his way back to the bathroom when the doorbell rang.

'Is that Mr Philip Fletcher?' said the crackly voice on the intercom. Philip admitted that it was. 'I've a delivery for you.'

'Leave it inside the front door, please.'

'I need a signature.'

'First floor.'

He pressed the button reluctantly. It was as well that he had scraped off the make-up, but he was still wearing women's underwear beneath his dressing gown, and nothing else. He went quickly to the bedroom to take off his stockings, a fiddly business. He heard a loud hammering next door.

'Hang on!' he muttered, hurrying back to the living room. He seized the handle and pulled it back a couple of inches. 'Where do you want me to –'

The door was flung open violently in his face, catching him a stinging blow on the nose. He staggered back, lost his balance and fell against the sofa. He was much too stunned to say anything as two men dressed in black over-coats walked into his front room and closed the door behind them.

'Aw, sorry about that,' said the smaller and older of the two men. 'Mr Lewis here don't know his own strength sometimes. Give Mr Fletcher a hand up, will you, Mr Lewis?'

Philip said nothing as Mr Lewis, a cross between Bluto and the Wild Man of Borneo, grabbed his lapels and yanked him to his feet.

'I hope he didn't break nothing,' said his friend in a concerned voice. 'You're not to break nothing, all right? Now, help Mr Fletcher to a seat.'

Still holding the dressing gown lapels tightly in his fists, the primate half lifted and half dragged Philip across the carpet before flinging him into his armchair. Although indignation was beginning to oust astonishment, Philip was still too disoriented to give his outrage voice. He did, however, attempt instinctively to rise. Mr Lewis promptly socked him on the jaw.

'Tut! Tut!' said the other man. 'I do hope he ain't broken nothing, Mr Fletcher. But if he has, you've only yourself to blame.'

The punch in the face had at last driven Philip over and way beyond the threshold of amazement. From having been in a sustained whirl for the last half-minute, his brain became suddenly focused. No one had hit him since child-hood. He wasn't by nature a scrapper, he neither expected to thump or be thumped. He registered the throbbing in his cheek, but was pleasantly surprised that it hadn't hurt more. In the movies a blow like that was usually enough to lay a man out.

'Now, all I want's a little talk, Mr Fletcher,' said the smaller man, in his infuriatingly paternalistic tone. He sat down across from him on the arm of the sofa. 'Just have the goodness to listen up, and there'll be no need for any more physical stuff, all right?'

The man was about Philip's age, slightly shorter but rather pudgier. An air of general unwholesomeness hung over him. It was apparent in the sweaty, glistening face, the small watery eyes, the thick flabby lips. The fingers which he brushed with an almost fastidious touch through his few but overlong dark hairs were darkly stained with nicotine. It was easy to see why he employed Mr Lewis to do his dirty work.

'Now,' the man continued, 'I expect you're wondering why I'm here –'

'Is my council tax overdue?' Philip suggested.

'I hope that's not your idea of a joke, Mr Fletcher. I shouldn't like to have to ask my friend here to get physical again. No, that's not why I've come –'

'Then I expect Doris sent you.'

The flicker of annoyance at the second interruption told Philip he was on the right track. Not that it had been difficult to guess.

'Now this'll be over a lot quicker, Mr Fletcher, if you just sit quiet and stop sticking your oar in, all right? I am, as you have so rightly, and cleverly, surmised, an associate of a certain individual, of a kind what is commonly called a "character", if you get my drift. Horses for courses, I say, different strokes for different folks. Not for me to judge, and Mr Lewis here will confirm that I'm as broad-minded as the next bloke. What people gets up to in the privacy of their own homes is their business, as long as they don't expect to include me in it. I'm not in that line myself, and nor, if I may hazard a guess, are you. But that's not the point. Doris is a friend, and I do not like to see friends of mine getting hassled. Now that's all very well and good, you might say. What do I care, you might go on to ask, if that Mr Dorigo fellow (that's me, by the way – sorry we weren't properly introduced) has expressed displeasure and disquiet at my behaviour? Well, if it was just me I could understand your position, but it ain't, you see. My associate here, Mr Lewis, he's a bit of a loose cannon, I'm afraid. Very fond of his friends, he is, and Doris is a particular chum, though don't go thinking he's a shirt-lifter himself, he wouldn't take kindly to that sort of suggestion and he's not as tolerant as I am. Do you get what I'm saying, Mr Fletcher? If you will insist on mucking that certain individual about I cannot be responsible for Mr Lewis's actions. He's liable to get a bit, well, you know . . .'

'Physical?' Philip suggested.

'Took the word out of my mouth. I'm glad to see we understand each other. You're an actor, aren't you, Mr Fletcher?'

'I am.'

'I seen you on the box. I'm a big fan of yours, and the missus, she is too. She said to me on more than one occasion, "oh, I could fancy that Philip Fletcher, I could".'

'How flattering.'

'It's no more than your due. You're a handsome feller, quite the ladies' man, I daresay. But it wouldn't be the same for you, I'm afraid, if my friend here was to rearrange your face, as he has been known to do from time to time to people that get on his tits. As I say, Mr Fletcher, I am a tolerant man, but I do have standards and I have to be strict. With me there's no such thing as a final warning. This is it, it's your first warning, and it's your one and only. Sorry about this, but Mr Lewis – will you kindly demonstrate the point?'

Mr Lewis had been hovering behind the armchair, a menace felt but unseen. He appeared suddenly in front of Philip, seized him again by the lapels and dragged him up. It would have been fruitless to resist, and he didn't try. Instead he braced himself.

'Not the face, please, Mr Lewis.'

The second punch was a short hard jab to the solar plexus. It was much more painful than the first blow, it winded Philip and doubled him up in a heap on the carpet. The heavy put a foot on his shoulder and pushed him over on to his back.

'Well, well, Mr Fletcher,' said Mr Dorigo drily. 'I'd never have guessed!'

Philip felt himself redden. The dressing gown had slipped open, revealing his choice of Marks and Spencer matching black lace bra and suspender set. The heavy lifted back a foot ready to kick him.

'That'll do, Mr Lewis. There's enough gratuitous violence on the telly every night without us making a contribution. Go and keep an eye on the car, will you?'

'You be all right?' said the heavy thickly, opening his mouth for the first time. The effort it cost him seemed out of proportion to the eloquence of the sentiment expressed.

'Yeah, yeah, this one's a powder puff. I'm more worried about the car. Now push off.'

Philip didn't know whether to feel relieved at the big thug absenting himself, or mortified to find himself considered so unthreatening. He sat up against the armchair, nursing his wounded stomach, but unable to salve his pride. When his friend had left, Mr Dorigo resettled himself more comfortably on the arm of the sofa.

'It's a bugger finding a meter round here, you know,' he said pleasantly, taking cigarettes and a lighter out of his overcoat pocket.

'I'm surprised you bother about things like that,' muttered Philip irritably. He wasn't feeling in the mood for social chitchat.

'Aw, Mr Fletcher, I think you got me wrong. I pays my taxes, I'm an ordinary citizen, a businessman, and that's why I've asked young Mr Lewis to leave us for a minute, while we have a bit of a supplementary. He's a good lad, heart of gold beneath that bluff exterior, lovely to his mum, you should see them together, gives you a glow all over, but he's not got a head for detail, and frankly, I don't like to have him around when I'm discussing the old minutiae. You don't mind if I smoke, do you?'

He didn't wait for an answer, but lit up anyway.

'Aw, that's better! Now, the thing is, I don't mind mentioning Doris's name in front of Mr Lewis, but the actual precise nature of the business is delicate and private and that is how I wish to keep it, under wraps, you with me? Now Doris says you've been acting off your own bat, a bit of private enterprise, very laudable in its way, I admire the old entrepreneurial spirit myself, but, and this is the big but, Philip, my friend, if you'll allow me to get familiar for a minute, BUT this is the point where your involvement gets strangled at birth, you with me? I understand you haven't breathed a dickeybird to anyone about this, not even, and especially not even, to a certain young man closely related to what you might call the principal in this case, and for whom you have been acting as a go-between. I hope sincerely for your sake that this is the case. Now listen carefully, because as I have already made clear I never repeat myself. You are to cease all contact with that aforementioned young gentleman forthwith; the names of Doris, me, or anyone else connected with the case are not to be uttered or even so much as thought of, and, if I was you, speaking candidly and on an off-the-cuff basis, I'd make myself scarce for a while. Take a holiday. Go and lie on a sun-kissed beach for a fortnight. It'd be better than finding yourself lying face down in a deserted quarry, which I'm afraid to say is the only other option seriously on offer if you carry on sticking your nose in where it's not wanted. There, that's all, I'm done. It's a lot better, you see, if you just keep your trap shut and listen. Now all it remains for me to do is to say thank you for giving me some of your valuable time, and I'll be on my way. When can we expect the pleasure of seeing you again on the TV, Mr Fletcher? It's been a while, hasn't it?'

Philip did not feel inclined to discuss his career with his unwelcome visitor. He said nothing.

'Not feeling too bright, eh?' said Mr Dorigo from the door. 'I understand. Oh, and don't worry, your secret's safe with me. I know a lot of blokes like to dress up in women's gear, doesn't mean nothing at all. By the way, if you do decide to get away, I can recommend Portugal. The Algarve's deserted this time of –'

He was interrupted by the sound of the door buzzer. He stared at the intercom with some surprise.

'I hope that's not another delivery for you, Mr Fletcher,' he chuckled. 'Two in one day'd be a bit much. Stay where you are, I'll get it. Hello?'

Mr Dorigo winked at Philip and put the entry phone to his ear. In an instant the slimy grin evaporated from his face.

'Shit!' he swore, flinging down the receiver and rushing over to the window. 'I don't believe it!'

He turned back into the room with clenched teeth and knitted brow.

'Pardon me, Mr Fletcher.'

Angrily he pulled a mobile phone from his coat pocket and stabbed out some numbers.

'Dave, it's Vincent. I'm in Highbury Terrace, N5. The sodding car's been clamped again . . . I know, I only left it for five minutes, the bastards . . . Yeah, you'll sort it out, will you? Much obliged . . . Yeah, it's at the top of Highbury

Crescent, junction of Ronalds Road . . . No, no, I'll get a cab back. Cheers.'

He thrust the phone back into his pocket. He was wearing a look of supreme disgust.

'Don't know what the country's coming to,' he muttered, half to Philip, half to himself. 'It's a bloody liberty, if you ask me. Good afternoon, Mr Fletcher.'

He exited in a huff, leaving the front door wide open. Philip had to go over and close it. Then he stumbled next door and collapsed on to his bed.

He felt utterly enervated. He was used to people illicitly gaining entry to his flat, but assault and battery marked a worrying departure from the norm. Not that he had been hurt badly, but it was the thought that counted. Events were getting seriously out of hand.

So what should he do now? The sensible option would be to quit and cut his losses. The warning shot across his bows had been unsubtle and unambiguous. Mr Dorigo and his cerebrally challenged friend may have cut rather absurd figures, but Philip didn't suppose for a moment that the threats had been idle. If he crossed Doris and his shady pals again he'd have more to reckon with than the odd punch. They knew where to come and find him. His address, he presumed, they had found in Seymour's diary.

He did some breathing exercises, tensed and relaxed his muscles, tried to calm down. His pulse steadied, but he could feel a headache developing. He went to the bathroom to look for some aspirin.

He took two, finished the glass of water, then poured another and drained it thirstily. His throat was dry, the rest of him still moist with sweat. But the tension had gone. He examined his face in the mirror. The side of his jaw was a little red, but it didn't hurt. His teeth were all firmly in place.

'Powder puff indeed . . .'

If that was the hardest Mr Lewis could hit then perhaps

the soubriquet should be reapplied. He smiled mirthlessly at his reflection.

'I don't think they know who they're dealing with, do they?'

He imagined Vincent Dorigo telling it how it was to Doris and Norman. How he thought it was . . . Oh yeah, sorted that poovy actor feller out all right. Put the frighteners on him a treat. He's just a poncy theatrical type, you won't get no bother from him. A powder puff . . .

Philip's cold smile tightened. The phrase rankled. Who did they think they were, bursting into his flat, intimidating and threatening him, poking fun at his choice of underwear? He wasn't afraid of them. He'd dealt with their sort before, and dealt with them pretty effectively. He may have underestimated the opposition in the present case, but by jingo they'd underestimated him too.

'They just have no idea, do they? They might have brute force and ignorance on their side, but I have cunning, talent, brains, and a mastery of disguise unequalled in the roll-call of British Equity. And if you lot think you're going to come between me and my just deserts, you've got another think coming . . .'

It was just as well they hadn't cut or bruised his face, he had a performance to prepare. Several performances, to be precise. The big one would be tomorrow night, and required much more detailed preparation than he had thus far given it. He stripped, lathered up his shaving brush and began applying his razor to his body.

He'd never thought of himself as hirsute, but now he looked closely he seemed to have stray hairs everywhere. He shaved his arms and armpits, his neck and shoulders and chest down to the bra line. The legs took longest. When he had finished he felt like a plucked chicken. Once in the bath he covered his eyes with his flannel, partly as an aid to concentration, partly so that he wouldn't have to look at himself. What exactly was this Marlene von Trapp about? Was he a man pretending to be a woman, but knowing full well that he wasn't? Or was the illusion meant to be more than skin-deep? With role-models as diverse as Doris Afternoon and Melanie Mockingbird it was hardly surprising that he felt confused.

He dried himself briskly and dressed, with relief, as himself again. It was mid-afternoon, he supposed he ought to eat something, but he felt too nervous for food. He picked up the phone and ordered another cab. The day had gone by in a rush, from the morning audition, the return to his hotel (where he'd paid for a week in advance; he still had the room-key and an alternative bolt-hole), thence to Conchita's flat and back in time for his interview with Mr Dorigo. He would have liked a nap, but he simply had too much to do. He allowed himself a small Scotch as a pick-me-up. What he really wanted was a cigarette; he felt an intense regressive craving. Just as well he didn't have any, he thought wryly to himself, then noticed to his horror that twenty Bensons and a lighter were sitting on the arm of the sofa. Not content with assaulting him physically, Vincent had compounded the offence by leaving dread temptation in his way. For ten minutes, until the cab came, Philip sat staring at the shiny gold packet, a victim of brutal psychological torture. At last the buzzer rang.

'All that glisters is not gold,' he told himself pitifully, as he left the packet on the hall table. The cheap disposable lighter he hung on to, like a comfort blanket. He snatched up his briefcase and raced downstairs.

He ordered the taxi to take him to Knightsbridge. As they turned out of Highbury Terrace he noted a large silver Volvo parked on the corner, the front wheel obscured by a yellow Denver boot. If it was still there when he came back he might let down the tyres. The thought consoled him on the tedious journey through thick traffic. He sat

127

fiddling with the lighter and tried to take his mind off nicotine by dreaming of revenge.

His destination lay just behind Harrods. He approached the intercom, and, after a long moment's scrutiny by the security cameras, was admitted through the black steel door. A uniformed receptionist studied his identification, checked with a computer, then spoke into a phone.

'John, will you come and take Mr Fletcher downstairs, please?'

An electric buzzer sounded and an inner door clicked open. Philip went in.

'Good afternoon, sir. This way, please.'

Philip followed the guard into the lift and they went down one floor to the basement. They stepped out into a narrow corridor, blocked at the end by an imposing metal grille. As they approached, another uniformed guard appeared on the other side and unlocked it.

'To the right, sir,' he said, indicating a door.

Philip knew the way. He went through the plain steel door and the guard closed it after him, leaving him alone in the low-ceilinged room. The safe deposit boxes were stacked in rows, like left-luggage lockers. His own, which he hadn't visited for months, was halfway down on the left.

He found it and inserted a long slim key. The lock clicked open smoothly. Philip tucked his briefcase under his arm, pulled out the rectangular metal box within and carried it over to one of the tables in the corners. Opaque plastic partitions fixed to the tables ensured extra privacy.

In the box were two plastic carrier bags. One of them contained a wooden cigar box. The other was crammed full of cash.

Methodically, Philip took out all the money and stacked it on the table. He didn't need to, in fact it was a complete waste of time, but he was enjoying himself. The money was bundled in wads of twenty- and ten-pound notes, 'used and untraceable' as they always said in the movies and as he had said to Ken Kilmaine. An actor to his finger-tips, it was his nature never to use his own lines if someone else's would do.

There were twenty bundles of twenties, one hundred notes and two thousand pounds in each. He transferred two to his briefcase, and took one of the thirty-two remaining bundles of tens, another thousand pounds. That left £67,000 out of the hundred grand he had so successfully extracted from the deceased and unmissed film producer. He supposed that it ought really to be sitting in a Swiss bank account somewhere (Switzerland, perhaps), but he liked the idea of having a safe deposit box, it made him feel important as well as stimulatingly shady, whereas a Swiss account would have just made him feel common and shady. Furthermore, he was less interested in hoarding the money than in spending it, that seeming to him the purpose for which it had been devised. Knightsbridge was rather more convenient than Zurich.

And he would have needed the safe deposit box anyway, to take care of the second item. When he had had enough of playing with the stack of money he put it away, and turned his attention to the cigar box. As he opened the lid a thick mattress of paper tissue sprang up. He removed it carefully and took out the gun with which Shelley Lamour had tried to kill him.

It was a small, black-handled Smith & Wesson revolver, a neat little .38 with a two-inch barrel. It fitted comfortably into the hand, or into the handbag, an ideal ladies' gun. In fact, it was called a LadySmith. It was compact and lightweight, but had excellent stopping power. It said all this, and more, in the brochure he had ordered from America. He was glad that Shelley had not had a chance to test its stopping power properly. The one bullet she had fired had merely nicked his leg.

There were five cartridges still in the chamber. He took

them out, weighed and played with them, admiring the silvery glint of the bullets, the duller brass gleam of the cases. He replaced them, snugly. He had oiled the gun on his last visit, following instructions in a book, and it appeared to be in smooth working order. He imagined pointing it at Doris and his friends.

Vincent Dorigo would be surprised. What, that poovy actor? A tooled up powder puff? For the threat to be valid it would have to be backed up by clear intention, and he had never shot anyone in his life. Handguns were notoriously inaccurate. What if he missed? He imagined Doris's bulk looming before him, a target of barn-door proportions. It would actually be harder to miss than to hit. As for pulling the trigger, he had only to think of the humiliating going-over he'd just received for the prospect of planting a bullet smack between the eyes to become instantly and wildly appealing.

He hesitated. He had come for the money, but he'd made his plans before the visit from Vincent Dorigo. It looked as if the rules of the game had been revised. Firearms were not in his province, but he might need all the insurance he could get. It could be a very useful prop. Just how badly did he want Seymour's diary? He thought about it for a moment and decided that the answer was very badly. He put the gun back into the cigar box and transferred it to the briefcase. Then he locked up and left.

He walked out into the late-afternoon darkness, clutching the heavy briefcase to his chest. He hoped, for their sake, that no one tried to mug him. He might be a powder puff to some, but he was beginning to feel like Rambo.

He picked up a cab in Knightsbridge and headed back to Highbury. He'd do some essential packing, then seal up his flat and disappear for as long as it took. For all anyone could know or care, Philip Fletcher had gone to the Algarve. There would be nothing to link him with a female impersonator currently resident in Cumberland Mansions, and for emergencies he still had the hotel room in Bays-water, although he could live comfortably without the sniggers of the hall porter. His life was complicated enough already without inviting further intrusions from Vincent Dorigo and his ilk.

As the cab turned into Highbury Terrace, Philip noted that the silver Volvo was still parked on the corner. On an impulse he walked back down the road to inspect it.

The clamp had actually been removed. Perhaps Mr Lewis was even now en route to reclaim possession. He'd better be quick if he was going to let down the tyres. On mature reflection, childish pranks did not appeal. He peered through the windows. Some dark material, it might have been a coat, lay across the back seat. Philip wondered if there were anything interesting in the pockets.

Had George been around he could have found out. George could break into cars in his sleep; the waking hours he reserved for domestic burglary. Cars were the easiest job in the world, the boy always said. Half the time owners didn't even know they were born. It was amazing how often they didn't even remember to lock the doors.

Philip tried the off-side doors; no luck. He walked round to the driver's side, waited for a pedestrian to go by, then tried again. It didn't budge. Clearly Mr Lewis did know that he'd been born. Then again, it was perhaps the only thing he did know.

Philip hesitated. He drummed out a little contemplative beat on the roof of the car, then trailed his finger down the rear window and the boot as he walked slowly round the back. His finger brushed over the button lock. Idly he pressed it in, and heard a dull click. The boot was open. Either someone had been very careless or the central lock-ing wasn't functioning. He glanced around to check that no one was looking, then lifted the lid and propped it open.

No light came on. He patted the bottom of the boot with his hands and felt his way around the spare tyre. He had no idea what he was looking for – nothing probably, it was just nosiness; curiosity; chancing. His fingers came into contact with a metal box. He felt in vain for a catch. He remembered that he had Vincent Dorigo's lighter in his pocket.

He flicked it on and examined the box. The catch was at the top, fiddly and difficult to open. Eventually he managed it. The box was full of tools. He turned the wheel on the lighter until he could make a fearsome five-inch flame and waved it into the corners. The boot was empty.

'Anything the matter, sir?' said a friendly voice behind him.

Philip jumped, banging his head on the boot lid. Bloody typical, he thought, as his eyes adjusted again to the street-light and he made out the details of the policeman's uniform; there's always one around when you don't need one.

'Oh, nothing, thanks, officer,' he lied haltingly. 'Just thought I'd dropped something, that's all. The boot light's broken.'

'Lucky I'm here, then, sir. I've got a torch.'

Bully for you, thought Philip, setting his teeth into a grim clench. He tried to avert his face from the torchlight.

'Now what was it you dropped, sir?'

'A pen,' said Philip smoothly, having recovered his natural gift for fluent fabrication.

'Ah yes, here it is!'

Philip couldn't have been more surprised at the sight of the black plastic biro being held up for his inspection. He took it, though, and put it in his pocket.

'Thank you so much, officer,' he said, gushing relief. 'I don't know what I'd have done without you.'

'Don't mention it, sir, I'm happy to oblige.' The police-man chuckled. 'We're not all bastards, you know!'

'I didn't suppose for a moment that you were. Good night, officer.'

'Good night, sir.'

The policeman actually touched his helmet with his forefinger. As he walked away down the street, Philip could have sworn that he heard him whistling to himself. George Dixon would have been proud.

Philip had lost all interest in the car. He just wanted to get home. As soon as the policeman had disappeared from view, he dropped the boot lid back into place and scarpered down the street.

He was still trembling twenty minutes later, even after a large refortifying whisky. He stood nervously by the door, his hastily packed suitcase on the floor beside him, waiting for the minicab he'd just ordered, the last in a long day. Twice he'd had Vincent Dorigo's cigarette packet in his hands; once he'd even had a filter to his lips. If he'd been able, at that moment, to find the lighter, he probably would have succumbed, but it didn't seem to be in his pocket any longer. He must have dropped it when the policeman had startled him. Had he been a more superstitious sort, he might have considered the whole episode providential. When at length the intercom buzzed he summoned up a supreme last-ditch effort and left the packet of cigarettes where he had found it.

He had set the alarm and double-locked everything in sight. The answerphone was set, the heating switched right down. Philip Fletcher, it appeared, was about to take Vincent Dorigo's advice and disappear. He asked the minicab driver to take him to Cumberland Mansions.

11

'You've got five minutes, Miss von Trapp,' said Sandy, putting his head round the dressing room door.

Philip murmured a dry inaudible thank you, but Sandy had already gone. He wondered when he was going to get his voice back. He'd never felt so nervous in his life.

Not all the terrors of all the first nights of his career rolled into one quivering ball of anxiousness could compete with this. It was as well he'd spent an hour on his make-up before setting off – he couldn't have held his eyebrow pencil steady for long enough to sketch a straight line. It was a relief that Sandy had been on hand to zip him up.

A relief, too, that he was alone. Doris would be in later, Sandy had warned him, which he found a disquieting prospect. The dressing room was so tiny he didn't see how they'd both fit in. Already Doris's costumes, a vomiting kaleidoscope of silks and taffeta, took up most of the available space. Engulfed on all sides by swathes of outsize colour-uncoordinated clothing, Philip felt like a one-man safari lost in an Oxfam shop.

At least, he reflected, staring at his bizarre reflection in the mirror, his disguise was impenetrable. Neither his nor anyone else's mother would have recognized him. He was used to the distorting effects of make-up, but this transformation astonished even himself. He only hoped his acting skills would revive in time to do it justice. His singing skills alone were unlikely to see him through.

He closed his eyes, breathed deeply, tried to relax. Tension was even more of an enemy to a singer than to an actor, and he was tenser than a suspension bridge. He went over some lyrics in his head. He hadn't had time to learn Lili Marleen. He'd fallen back on 'Mack the Knife' for his second number because it was thematic as well as familiar, easy. At least it had appeared so at the time, in the cool of a private one-on-one lesson with his arranger friend. Why couldn't he remember it now? What on earth happened in the middle passage? It'll just come, he told himself, attempting to summon a philosophical disposition; it'll be all right on the night.

'Miss von Trapp!' called Sandy through the door. 'You're on!'

Shit! thought Philip. This *is* the night . . .

The background buzz coming through the tannoy swelled in his head. Feeling giddy, he stood before the full-length mirror by the door and gave himself one last despairing look. Was that a natural shimmer in the metallic blue of his dress, or was it just him shaking?

He opened the door and stepped out gingerly into the corridor, balancing awkwardly on his disconcerting heels. To his left was the fire exit that led up to the lobby and street level; he could hear the sirens cooing to him from the pavement. Yes, he could still run, but then he couldn't come back. He thought of his reasons for being there in the first place, and steeled himself. He turned the other way.

The stairs that led up to Doris's office were behind him now; the curtain masking the entrance to the club dead ahead. Norman was holding an edge of the material and peering out. When he saw Philip he nodded to someone on the other side.

'Good house tonight,' he announced curtly. 'I'll play you an intro, like we rehearsed, then get your arse on stage quick and start singing. No chitchat, Doris doesn't like it.'

Norman disappeared through the curtain.

'And good luck to you, too,' Philip murmured drily under his breath.

It hadn't been much of a rehearsal. Norman had spent most of the ten minutes or so allotted to grumbling about the fact that Philip wasn't going to sing Lili Marleen. Philip had had to be very firm with him. The stricter he was, he had confirmed, the more malleable Norman became.

'Ladies and gentlemen!' boomed the microphoned voice of the compere on the other side of the curtain, and, after a pause: '. . . and those who aren't quite sure . . .'

Whistles and laughter sang out in response. It sounded like a healthy crowd, as promised.

'Tonight we have a very special treat for you!' declared the compere.

'Oooh!' answered the audience.

'No, no, not him!' said the compere, with mock-disgust. 'You'd have to be a major sort of a perve to regard old Norman as any kind of a treat!'

'Aaah!' answered some of the audience, with mock-sympathy. Norman-baiting was obviously a well-established sport.

'No, no!' continued the compere. 'It's a genuine international treat we have for you tonight. Will you please put your hands together and extend the warmest of Bosie Butterflys very special welcomes to that international artiste and glittering star of the Heidelberg cabaret, the one and only, the inimitable fantasy fräulein herself, Miss Marlene von Trapp!'

Oh, that this too too solid flesh would melt! Philip thought to himself. He stiffened the sinews and summoned up the blood; he'd already stepped out of his breeches.

He dropped the curtain behind him and stepped on to the translucent pink stage. Bright lights and applause flooded over him. He was blinded by the sharp white profile spots, but he could sense the crowd, feel them, smell them – the basement air was thick with condensed sweat and sweet perfumes. A chorus of wolf-whistles greeted him as he reached the microphone stand.

'Danke schön!' he breathed sensuously into the microphone, fluttering his improbably long false lashes. 'You certainly know how to make a girl feel velcome!'

Members of the audience were shouting comments at him in response. He couldn't make them out, but he smiled and nodded knowingly. A brisk impatient tinkle from Norman reminded him of his obligations – no chitchat, he was here to warble. He acknowledged the pianist with a casual wave, and Norman immediately launched himself into the intro to 'Moon of Alabama'.

Whether it was because of nerves or lack of rehearsal Philip was never sure, but he came in a good beat late on cue, and never recovered. By the end of the first verse he was trailing hopelessly, but the further he fell behind the faster Norman seemed to play. Philip's vision blurred. In the dry silence he could hear the thumping of his pulse, the gasps for air that still left him hopelessly short of breath, and fancied that he heard them amplified back at him over the sound system. The performer's worst nightmare, disintegration, was staring him in the face. The audience had gone deathly quiet.

He stopped singing. Norman carried on, all the way through the first chorus, at the end of which he brought himself to a gradual reluctant halt. Philip could feel the murderous eyes boring through him, but he didn't glance aside. He stood looking straight ahead, serenely cool. The unqualified completeness of his failure had taken him above and beyond mere panic. He felt really rather detached.

And odder still, he felt in control. He could sense the audience's restlessness, their embarrassment on his behalf, but at the same time he sensed their focus, too. Every eye was fixed on him, every breath caught and surprised in aspic in the collective throat. He experienced a surge of unimagined and unimaginable raw confidence.

This is more like it, he told himself with perverse satisfaction. Sod that singing lark, this is *theatre* . . .

'Vell, vell,' he drawled into the microphone, when the last exasperated note from the piano had died away. He raised a supercilious eyebrow and turned his most disapproving gaze at Norman: 'Vat's the big idea, munchkin? Vat kind of drugs are you on?'

A nervous semi-titter came from the audience. They were uncertain, but still aching to be convinced.

'I don't take drugs!' hissed Norman, his rodent features stretched white with fury.

'Mein Gott!' gasped Philip. 'You mean you're not ze result of some hideous laboratory experiment gone vrong?'

Philip let his eyes bulge and turned to share his amazement with the audience. The titters grew full-blown.

'What's your problem, then?' Norman spluttered, but his thin unamplified voice had little impact. Philip almost caressed the microphone with his lips.

'My problem, sveetie, iss having a dummkopf like you for an accompanist. Vere did you learn? Ze London school for ze deaf?'

Norman's outraged response was drowned in a burst of spontaneous applause. Philip wagged a reproachful finger at him.

'Ach! I ought to bend you over your piano and spank some sense into you, you naughty, naughty boy!'

Norman turned bright red at the suggestion.

'Und zat's a threat, baby,' Philip added sternly, 'not a promise.'

'After him, please!' called out a bold masochist from the back of the audience.

'You'll have to join ze queue,' said Philip teasingly. He noticed Norman, his complexion changing rapidly between crimson and puce, attempting to rise from his stool. 'Vere do you think you're going, schweinhund?'

Philip cracked the flex of his microphone like a lion tamer. Norman recoiled, like a kitten. An awed whisper drifted over from the audience:

'Blimey, it's Miss von Whiplash!'

'Sit!' commanded Philip magisterially. Norman sat. 'Gut boy! On ze count of three you vill play "Moon of Alabama", und zis time you vill get it right or zere vill be big trouble, you know vat I mean? Ein, zwei, drei!'

Snap! went the flex, and bang! went the ivories. Philip hurled himself into the song with manic abandon, and this time it was Norman who struggled to keep up. The audience loved it. When he got to the line about finding the next little boy, a whole row of them appeared at the front of the stage, big eyes plaintively wide and dry mouths slackly open. One dared to caress the toe of Philip's shoe. The look of withering contempt he got for his pains sent him into transports of ecstasy.

The applause at the end was volcanic. Punters at the back were standing on their seats to get a better look. At the front the whooping crowd was pressed tight against the stage, no doubt to the discomfort of some but to the delight of a great many more. Enough flowers to denude a fair-sized English country garden were tossed at Philip's feet.

After a minute or so of basking in adoration Philip felt the applause begin to wane. He also noticed Norman trying to say something to him from the piano. Philip gave his flex another sharp little flick.

'Cut out ze chitchat, baby, just play!'

Norman did as he was bid. Huskily sinister, Philip gave his 'Mack the Knife'. The violent imagery, which he stressed to the hilt, sent his lesser-hearted listeners into protective huddles. His eyes long since adjusted to the light, he made out Melanie and Rita holding each other's hands for support. They were both wide-eyed with admiration.

139

The applause for his second number was a little more muted, but no less heartfelt. The air was filled with cries of 'Encore!' Philip shook his head firmly.

'Nein, zat's enough for now. I don't vant to spoil you.'

Leave them wanting more, he'd always been taught. Besides, he didn't know anything else.

He exited imperiously, with thunderous clapping in his ears and a freshly donated bouquet of carnations held to his padded bosom. Sandy held the curtain aside for him.

'Fantastic, Miss von Trapp, could I have your autograph?'

'Later sveetie, for now I vant to be alone.'

His Marlene promiscuously eliding into a Greta, he grandly re-entered the dressing room, where, unfortunately, his desire for solitude was rudely thwarted.

'What the fuck was that all about then?' demanded Doris Afternoon harshly.

Doris was sitting in semi-undress in front of the mirror, his vast corseted frame flowing over the tiny wooden chair provided. He looked like an elephant perched on a toadstool. Philip saw very little prospect of being able to squeeze past and get at his own clothes.

'I beg your pardon?' he responded coolly from the door.

'You heard. What was that crap you were giving Norman then? You want to work here again, love, you just get out there and do the old songbird routine. The jokes and the chat you leave to me, all right?'

'Ah, ja?' said Philip, seething but trying to sound unruffled. 'Anyzing else?'

'Yes, you can knock off that dumb phoney German accent when you're offstage. It's called overegging the pudding.'

'Ooh, ve are in a bad mood tonight!'

'Cut it out, dear! I've met your sort before. I can see straight through you, and don't think I can't.'

Can't see through me quite as well as you think, Philip

140

thought. He hesitated. Unfortunately he couldn't afford to antagonize Doris. As much as it went against the grain, for now it would be sensible to feign penitence.

'I apologize if I have overstepped the mark,' he said quietly, lightening but not dropping his accent altogether.

'Well, don't do it again,' said Doris brusquely, turning back to the mirror and continuing with his make-up. He was already wearing enough to cater for an entire street of window displays in Amsterdam.

Sandy knocked on the door and poked his head round.

'Melanie and Rita wonder if you're coming out front, Marlene. They'd like to buy you a drink.'

'Please tell zem I vill be out shortly.'

With Doris in the room there wasn't really room for him to change, and in any case, his furtive and fertile brain sensed the glimmer of an opportunity. He'd be back later.

'I vonder if you'd be good enough to pass me my hand-bag, please?'

Reluctantly Doris put down his powder compact and passed over the bag.

'What you got in here then, love? It weighs a ton!'

Philip merely smiled.

'Gut luck, Miss Afternoon,' he said politely, and took his bag and left.

He went out not by the stage curtain, but by the fire exit, up the stairs to the entrance lobby. A push-bar meant that the door was always locked from the outside. Philip left it fractionally open (the doorman didn't notice), then went back down into the club by the main staircase.

Melanie and Rita had been sitting in one of the rear alcoves during his performance. They were still there. He slipped on to the padded bench next to them and gratefully took the proffered glass of white wine.

'Should be champagne really,' said Melanie apologetic-ally. 'You were magnificent!'

'Zis is fine,' said Philip. 'Tanks.' The wine at least was

drinkable, the champagne, he knew from experience, not so.

'I can't believe the way you dealt with Norman,' Melanie continued, sounding awestruck. 'I hope you heard us all raising the roof.'

Sandy appeared bearing a tray of exotic cocktails.

'From the gentleman on table seven,' he explained, leaving the drinks. 'With his compliments.'

Philip raised a milky fluted glass, adorned with miniature parasols and decorative cherries, in the direction of the table indicated. A soberly respectable middle-aged man in a pinstripe suit nodded back graciously.

'I'd watch him if I were you,' whispered Melanie urgently. 'He's a High Court judge, that one.'

'Kinky as hell,' chipped in Rita.

'Aren't zey all?' said Philip, knowingly. He tasted the drink, which was alcoholic and coconutty. 'Mm, not bad . . .'

'Sorry to bother you again,' said Sandy, reappearing. He handed Philip a single white rose. 'That's from table four, and this is from someone who asked me not to give his name . . .'

Sandy winked mysteriously and waltzed off again, leaving an unmarked white envelope on the table.

'You've made a big hit!' said Melanie.

The envelope contained a Polaroid photograph of a man's naked bottom, red with fresh weals. On the back was a phone number, and the message 'Please come up and see me some time!'

'Some vould like a bigger hit, I think,' Philip remarked, showing the photograph around. 'Anyone you know?'

Melanie and Rita giggled.

'Could be almost anyone in a place like this!' suggested Melanie. He nudged his friend. 'I think we should have a photo of our own, don't you?'

'Oh yes!' agreed Rita enthusiastically, taking a Polaroid camera out of his handbag. 'One for the record.'

A man sitting at the next table was prevailed upon to take a photograph of the three of them together. He said he would be delighted on condition that he could have a second one for himself.

'If Miss von Trapp would agree to sign it for me, please . . .' he added shyly.

Philip obliged with a grand flourish. The man seemed pleased with the picture but slightly disappointed with the autograph. Perhaps he'd hoped that Philip would leave his phone number too.

'Oh-oh!' said Melanie in a dramatic whisper. 'Don't look now, here comes trouble . . .'

Trouble meant Norman. He homed in on Philip like a heat-seeking missile.

'I wondered where the fuck you'd got to,' he said with his usual display of the social niceties.

'Just having a drink wiz my friends,' Philip answered defensively.

'Friends? Huh!'

Norman shot Melanie and Rita a withering glance. They withered.

'Why don't you two make yourselves scarce?'

'Come on, Rita,' whispered Melanie. 'Let's go and powder our noses . . .'

The two of them slid off the padded bench and scurried to the cloakrooms.

'You were enjoying yourself out there, then?' demanded Norman when they'd gone.

'Eventually, ja,' he responded curtly. 'Ven you got ze tempo right at last.'

'What do you mean? You were about a week late on cue!'

'Ha! Who are you kidding?'

'Look, fräulein, I've been at this game long enough to

143

know what's what, and you ballsed-up out there. But there's no need to get uppity, all right? I didn't come here to pick a fight with you.'

Norman smiled. Or rather he leered, hideously. Smiling didn't come naturally to him; the facial muscles had long ago fallen into desuetude.

'I want to compliment you, that's all. Your act went down a treat. I'd like us to be friends, Marlene.'

With awkwardly faked casualness Norman leant across the table and put his hand on Philip's knee.

'Real good friends, you know what I mean?'

Philip was afraid that he did. On reflection he had decided that he preferred Norman in his natural state of undiluted unpleasantness.

'Not so fast, mister. I'm not zat sort of a girl.'

'Oh, that's not what I've heard . . .'

Who on earth from? wondered Philip, as Norman's fingers began an unlicensed wander round his knee. He recovered himself in time to administer a sharp slap.

'Naughty, naughty boy!'

The harshness of the reprimand, alas, seemed only to encourage Norman's ardour. Fortunately, Philip's virtue was saved from compromise by the appearance of Sandy.

'Doris says ready when you are,' said the waiter to Norman, and to Philip: 'I've got a friend wants to meet you.'

'Ah, ja?'

'Here she is – Marcia, meet Marlene. Marlene, Marcia.'

A tall gaunt man in a carrot-coloured wig and silver lamé dress came and sat down next to Philip.

'Delighted to meet you, Marlene,' he said in a simpering Home Counties baritone. 'Hello, Norman.'

'Hello, Marcia,' answered Norman with a scowl. The smiling experiment seemed to be over for now, with normal service resumed. 'You'll have to excuse me, Doris is waiting. Catch you later.'

He gave Philip a meaningful glance as he departed. Loftily Philip ignored him.

'Such a sweetie, our Norman, isn't he?' suggested Marcia.

Philip gave the faintest of polite smiles.

'I was tremendously impressed by your performance, Marlene – do you mind if I call you Marlene? It's such an honour to meet you. A true artiste. There are a number of reputable theatrical agents in the club tonight. I shouldn't be surprised if one of them had noticed you.'

Philip had certainly noticed them. He carried on smiling blandly as Marcia suggested that he might well be able to swing a few introductions. It was not a career path he actually wished to explore.

'Ooh, who did *your* nails!' exclaimed Marcia suddenly, seizing his hand. 'What a lovely manicure! I can't do a thing with mine! They're awful, aren't they?'

He offered them for Philip's inspection. The fingers were oddly stubby, considering how long and thin the rest of him was, and the nails showed unmistakable signs of having been chewed. Philip quite agreed that they were awful, but he was too polite to say so.

'I'm sorry, you'll have to excuse me,' said Marcia, casting an eye at the stage. He edged off the padded seat, taking a portable phone out of his handbag. 'Just got to make a quick call. Catch you later, then!'

'Hope so,' Philip lied.

An exchange of girl-talk with a hairy-armed transvestite blue-jawed with five o'clock shadow was not his idea of fun. The rules of this gender-bending game were much too elastic for comfort. Where was the point of contact between someone like Melanie or Rita, so meticulously dolled up that at a penumbral distance they might easily be mistaken for women, and someone like Marcia, who at any distance and under any lighting conditions could only ever be taken exactly for what he was – a man in a dress? Who was kidding whom?

Norman had resumed his seat at the piano. Doris would be out any moment. Philip slipped out of the alcove and headed for the exit. As he climbed the stairs he heard the compere arrive on stage and begin his patter. As he went back through the artistes' door, left open as arranged, he heard Norman begin his intro. By the time he reached the dressing room Doris was belting out 'Somewhere Over the Rainbow'. He reckoned that he had about fifteen minutes.

He did a record-time quick change out of his evening gown and into his loose black skirt and blouse. He hung his costume up with his coat and his handbag on the only available hook, and joyfully exchanged high for flat heels. He riffled through Doris's personal effects, which were strewn over the table. In the handbag (an antique monstrosity in chain mail and diamanté) he found some keys, though not the one he sought. A big ugly bastard, George had told him to look out for. There was nothing to fit that description, but he took the bunch anyway.

He left the dressing room and climbed the office stairs. Through the curtain behind him he heard the muffled start of 'Nina from Argentina'.

He turned right at the top of the stairs, hurried down the landing. A single dim bulb lit the way. He turned right again, where the carpet gave out, walked along the bare squeaky floor to the bedroom door. It was locked. He fumbled with the bunch of keys, struck lucky at the second attempt. He pushed open the door, closed and locked it again behind him, and felt for the light switch.

The place was a tip. Discarded clothing littered the floor, mostly Doris's. More clothes seemed to be on the point of exploding from an overfilled and open wardrobe. A spilled wastebasket in the corner added its contents to the general slick, and even overflowed through the open bathroom door. The bed was unmade, the curtains undrawn. The wallpaper seemed to peel before his eyes.

But Philip had minimal interest in the decor. He walked in past the bed, noting drily the lengths of leather thong attached permanently to each of the legs. A chest of drawers caught his eye. He went through it, and found only more clothes. He turned his attention to the wardrobe. There was a big drawer at the bottom. He opened it, rummaged through a collection of whips, riding crops and assorted items of rubber and leatherwear. A couple of shoeboxes in the corner looked promising. He opened one, found only a pair of shoes. He heard a noise outside in the corridor, and held himself very still.

He didn't breathe. He sat crouched on his haunches, listening. Then he heard the noise again, the telltale squeak of a floorboard. A key rattled in the lock.

He could tell at a glance that the wardrobe wouldn't be big enough. He sprang up and dived through the bathroom door. He tried to shut it after him, but the rubbish on the floor meant it wouldn't close. Through the three-inch gap he saw the handle on the bedroom door turning. A moment later Mr Dorigo walked in.

From the furtive way he pocketed his skeleton key and glanced to left and right before reclosing the door, it was quite apparent that his presence was unauthorized. Philip backed off into the dark interior of the bathroom. Repositioning himself behind the door he found that he could see a little of the bedroom through the crack between the hinges. Mr Dorigo was examining the chest of drawers. When he had finished he approached the wardrobe. Philip could hear, but not see, him going through exactly the same routine he had just followed. It wasn't hard to guess what he might be looking for.

Honour among thieves, Philip reflected sagely. At another time he might have been amused. Unfortunately, his predicament was too severe for levity.

147

Doris would be finishing his act any minute now, while Philip was stuck upstairs where he shouldn't be in possession of a purloined set of keys. Uncomfortable memories flooded his brain. It wasn't the first time he'd been trapped in a bathroom.

The time slipped by. He couldn't see his watch, but he knew that Doris must be almost done. What if he came up and discovered first Mr Dorigo and then him? The bizarre scenario flashed across his imagination. He was jolted out of it by the shrill electronic bleep of a telephone going off next door.

Mr Dorigo appeared in view through the crack, hastily pulling a portable phone from his pocket.

'Yeah?' he whispered urgently into the receiver. There was a pause. 'Just finished? Yeah, yeah, I can hear the applause . . . nah, bugger all, dunno where it is . . . yeah, yeah, I'll be right down. Thanks, Marcia. Cheers.'

Mr Dorigo put the phone back in his pocket and gave the room a lingering disappointed look. He exited with a shrug. Philip could hear the noise of the key as he locked the door.

He waited till the squeaky floorboards were quiet again, then stared nervously at the second hand on his watch. He had to give Dorigo time to get away. If he bumped into him he'd say that he was looking for the bathroom. Lame, but Vincent was hardly in a position to challenge him, was he? He waited half a minute, then he used his own key on the door and bolted for it.

He ran as fast as he could along the carpetless corridor, the long landing, down the stairs. His heart sank. From halfway down he could hear Doris's voice. He sounded annoyed:

'. . . it's just not our sort of an act. We don't need anyone else, that's all there is to it.'

'Doris, you know bloody well we just can't get any decent quality at the moment,' Norman answered insistently. 'And you should hear the response I've been getting. The punters think she's terrific.'

What, little old me? wondered Philip with some bemusement. He was used to critics arguing publicly over his merits, but not the management. He would be sorry to break in on this little conversation, but he needed urgently to get into the dressing room. He turned the corner at the bottom of the stairs, and immediately bumped into Vincent Dorigo.

Vincent was skulking, there was no other word for it. It was obvious from his instantaneous change of complexion and the furtive way in which he clung to the wall that he'd been eavesdropping.

'Good evening, madam,' he said to Philip. He coughed to cover his confusion, then knocked on the dressing room door, which he was standing right next to, and which was an inch or so open.

'Oh, hello, Vince,' grunted Norman, when he'd stuck his head round to see who it was. 'Oh! Hello, Marlene!'

His unfamiliar grin split his mouth from ear to ear. He needed to keep practising. He looked like an auditionee for a Hammer Horror. Failed.

'Er, just arrived,' explained Vincent with another cough, though Norman wasn't paying him any attention. 'Er, has Marcus got here yet?'

He was trying extra hard to appear and sound innocent. Philip hadn't seen such bad acting since the last time he'd watched a prime-time mini-series.

'Lady Marcia's out front,' said Norman, his oily focus concentrated on Philip. 'So, Marlene, how you doing?'

'Vell, tanks. Excuse me, Norman, I haf to get into ze dressing room.'

'It's a bit crowded in there at the moment, dear. Why don't you get yourself a drink out front and pop back later?'

'Who's that?' demanded Doris crossly. He appeared behind Norman's shoulder.

'Blimey, it's like Piccadilly Circus!' joshed Vincent. Doris ignored him.

'What do you want?' he demanded of Philip.

'To get my handbag, if you vill excuse me –'

'I thought you'd already got your handbag?'

'I left it here again ven I came back to change.'

'Looks knockout, doesn't she?' exclaimed Norman. The filthy look he got in return was matched only by the one Doris was already giving Philip.

'Norman, take Vincent up to the office,' ordered Doris brusquely. 'Get him a drink. I'll get Marcia when I'm ready. Want my key?'

'I'm all right,' said Norman, patting his pocket. 'Oh, Marlene!'

'Ja?'

'Doris and I were just discussing how well you'd gone down tonight. We're hoping very much you'll be able to come back tomorrow and give us another set, aren't we, Doris?'

Doris didn't answer. Instead he just shot Norman a look which implied that he could expect extra special punishment tonight. Then he went back into the dressing room.

'I vould be honoured,' said Philip.

'Good. See you tomorrow afternoon, then. Same time. Come on, Vincent, let's go and get that drink . . .'

They walked away together, Norman waving some keys he'd just removed from his pocket. One of them was so big it barely fitted into his palm. Philip noticed that Vincent Dorigo seemed as interested in it as he was.

It distracted him for a moment from the rather more pressing key problem he had already. The bunch was clenched and sweaty in his fist. He held his hand behind his back as he re-entered the dressing room.

Doris was seated at the table removing some outer coats of face paint. The chain mail handbag was on the floor, exactly where it had been earlier.

'I wouldn't have given you a second chance myself,' said Doris icily, not taking his eye off the mirror. He dipped his pudgy fingers into a jar of face cream. 'Norman's too soft-hearted for his own good.'

'Ah, ja?'

It wasn't a description that would have sprung immediately to Philip's mind. He leant casually against the dressing room table.

'I vonder if I could get my coat and bag, Miss Afternoon – on ze hook behind you.'

Doris sighed crossly, swivelled on the stool and reached for the hook.

'Here!'

Philip took the bag and coat and lifted them over Doris's head. As he lowered them the coat tails caught the jar of cold cream and knocked it to the floor.

'Watch it, clumsy!' snapped Doris.

It was the work of a moment for Philip to kneel down and retrieve the jar with one hand, while the other, masked by his camel coat, casually dropped the bunch of keys into the maw of Doris's bag.

'Gut night, Miss Afternoon,' said Philip complacently, and left.

A masterful performance, he concluded to himself with no little satisfaction as he returned to the club room. Unfortunately he doubted that his other little difficulties could be overcome quite so easily.

'You're going, are you?' asked Melanie, indicating the coat slung over his arm.

'Ja, I am tired.'

'I'm not surprised! We'll come with you, share a cab. If you don't mind.'

'Nein, zat is . . . Melanie, I vonder if I might borrow your camera a moment. Hey, Marcia!'

Philip had just spotted the carrot-coloured wig. Its owner came gushing over like an old friend.

151

'Marcia, I vonder if I might have a snapshot, please, for my photograph album?'

Marcia was only too willing to oblige. He posed between Rita and Melanie, arms slung over their shoulders. Neither of them looked too happy about it, but they managed to strain a smile as the flashbulb went off.

'Not one of my favourites, that Marcia,' Melanie confided, as they left the club and walked out into the street. 'Too blowzy by half, if you ask me. Doesn't make a proper effort.'

'You should see her nails!' said Rita disapprovingly.

Philip had. They all stopped under a lamppost to pore over the developed photograph. Every aspect of Marcia's appearance came in for stinging criticism.

'Hello, darling!' shouted a semi-drunken youth from across the street.

'Can't see a cab anywhere,' muttered Rita nervously, pretending not to hear. 'Let's go this way.'

'Oi!' shouted out another youth. 'Give us a kiss!'

Philip followed Melanie and Rita northwards in the direction of the Marylebone Road. He was comfortable enough in his flat shoes, but the others both wore heels and long dresses and progress was slow. The streets were narrow and dark. Behind them they could hear footsteps, crisp and rapid on the pavement. By tacit agreement none of them glanced behind, just hoped that trouble would go away. It didn't.

There was a blur of movement as a figure ran past Philip's shoulder, then turned and stopped in front of them, blocking the pavement. Two more men came up, hemming them in from behind and to the side. They were outside a house lined with black iron railings.

'What we got here, then?' said the man at the front. There was no drunken slur in his voice now; only menace.

'Looks like some pansies in dresses,' sneered the one behind Philip. 'Hey, Ade, which one do you fancy?'

The one called Ade, who was a little older but even pimplier than the others, made a gagging noise.

'No, thanks.'

His friends took up his pantomime outrage and pretended to retch at the pavement.

'Excuse us,' said Melanie suddenly, his thin voice unexpectedly firm. 'We've got to be on our way now.'

He took Rita's hand and tried to walk on. Ade grabbed him by the throat and pushed him hard against the railings. Rita stifled a gasp of terror.

'Where you going, then?' demanded Ade, his right hand crushing Melanie's windpipe. In his left hand was a knife. The edge of the blade pressed hard into Melanie's neck. 'I ain't finished with you, you fucking pervert . . .'

'Stick him!' hissed one of the others gleefully, through gritted teeth.

Philip took his Smith & Wesson .38 out of his handbag and thrust it into Ade's face.

'Go on, asshole,' he said, as Dirty Harriet. 'Make my day!'

Ade appeared to be somewhat taken aback.

'He's bluffing!' said one of his friends after a moment of astonished silence, and then, less certainly: 'It's a fake!'

Philip pushed the barrel of the gun into the soft flesh of Ade's cheek.

'Try me,' he said calmly.

The day before he'd sat in the safe deposit room wondering if he'd ever have the nerve to pull the trigger. He knew the answer now. Ade must have known it too.

'Don't shoot!' he pleaded softly. 'I didn't mean nothing. Just a bit of fun, that's all.'

'Drop the knife,' said Philip.

The knife fell noisily to the ground.

'I would leave now, if I were you.'

Ade backed off, nervously. After a moment Philip lowered the gun, and, as if at a telepathic signal, the three youths simultaneously turned and ran for it. Philip put his gun back into his handbag.

'You were very brave,' he told Melanie. 'Let's go.'

Melanie and Rita followed him up the street. They were too stunned to speak. As they turned the next corner they spotted a cab.

'I'd be grateful if you didn't talk about this incident,' Philip said to them, when they had all settled themselves on the back seat.

'Oh no,' answered Melanie in a hoarse whisper. 'We won't.'

But even as he said it Philip must have known that he was wasting his breath. The already snowballing reputation of Marlene von Trapp, aka Miss von Whiplash, had just been swept up in an avalanche.

12

The first time Philip rang Sir Marcus Dalrymple he almost got through to the great man in person. The name he'd given, fictitious of course, had perhaps struck an unexpected chord. When he was told that Sir Marcus was on the other line and was asked to hold he agreed to do so, and then at once put down the phone.

When he rang back, half an hour later, he was told that Sir Marcus was at luncheon, which was where he should have been in the first place. Philip affected frustration and asked to be put through to his secretary.

'Hello, my dear,' he said to her in a familiar tone, 'it's Frank Walsingham. Done a bit of a boo-boo, I'm afraid. Made a note that I'd agreed to partner Marcus at bridge one afternoon this week, and blow me, can't read my own writing! You couldn't be an angel and check for me if it's today or tomorrow, could you?'

Not at all, said the secretary innocently. In fact, she didn't need to look at Sir Marcus's diary at all. He was on his way to the club even as they spoke. Frank Walsingham was immensely grateful to her.

As soon as he had put down the phone Philip went to the bathroom and began to work on his face. He wasn't planning a major job, more a character touch-up. He started by putting a dab of grey into the eyebrows, then ruddied his complexion with red grease-stick, subtly working his cheeks with blue to suggest a life at least partially misspent in lounge bars. He glued on a small precise moustache, the same shade as his refurbished brows. He oiled his hair and brushed it back, tight to the scalp. He took a small grey aerosol, shook it violently for a few moments, then applied a light even spray to the temples, brushing it through with his oily comb. He checked himself closely in the mirror and rubbed a stray fleck of grey paint from his forehead with the corner of his handkerchief.

Conchita's bathroom was well provided with mirrors. He paraded in front of them, examined himself from all angles. He was wearing a staid tweed suit that he'd bought years ago during a brief and misconceived *'Country Life'* phase. He'd only worn it once; it was comforting that it still fitted. He tried out three pairs of glasses and thought that none looked right. The idea of a monocle tempted him, but he knew it was over the top. He would go without. His disguise was hardly impenetrable, but it was adequate. He didn't expect to meet anyone he knew. Or at least, anyone who knew him.

The club the secretary had referred to was in Kensington. It was mentioned in a profile in last year's *Telegraph* (headed by a particularly severe photograph), which he'd obtained through his usual cuttings service. According to the newspaper, Sir Marcus was in the habit of playing there two afternoons a week, workload permitting, on the high-stakes table. It looked like he'd hit the bullseye with his first shot.

He checked the corridor outside the flat, then took the stairs down to the lobby. He encountered no one. He started to walk towards the Marylebone Road and soon picked up a cab. Ten minutes later he was in Kensington.

Despite the grand address, the building itself was in an unprepossessing state. The interior was nondescript, a sometime private residence which had simply acquired a function without a change of appearance. The room into which he wandered (there was no one around and the front door was unlocked) was a living room with a bar installed. An elderly couple were sitting in armchairs by the fire reading newspapers. They looked up eagerly when Philip came in.

'Are you here to play at the pound table?' asked the lady.

''Fraid not,' Philip replied.

The couple returned to their papers despondently. Philip approached the bar.

'Quiet this afternoon, eh?' he remarked to the barman.

He was told that there was a game on the five-pound table. He ordered a gin and tonic.

'Actually, I was rather hoping for something a touch spicier,' said Philip when he had received his drink. The barman looked dubious.

'Well, there is a twenty-pound table,' he admitted, 'but the standard's very high.'

'Sounds just the ticket!' said Philip grandly. 'Where do I sign up?'

He was given a book in which to register, offered club membership (which he declined) and charged a nominal fee as table money. He was directed upstairs, to the first floor, where he discovered a large and rather chilly room which contained half a dozen bridge tables. Only one was currently in use.

The four players seated round it were of markedly different ages and appearances, ranging from a vampirically pale young man in denims and earrings to a very frail old gentleman with spectacles so thick-lensed that he looked like a walking advertisement for a fairground hall of mirrors. The third player was a sharp-eyed bony matron who wore too much jewellery and much too much make-up. The fourth, currently the dummy, was Sir Marcus Dalrymple. He was the only one to look up as Philip approached.

'We've nearly finished the rubber,' said Sir Marcus

crisply, and turned his attention back to the play. He lit a cigarette.

The other three were puffing away already. Clouds of smoke swirled between the table and the ceiling. The green baize table stood like an altar at the heart of some arcane ceremony. As soon as the last card was laid down the ritual responses commenced.

'Why didn't you play on hearts?' demanded Sir Marcus.

'I was worried about the trump split,' answered the sharp-eyed lady. She had a slight middle-European accent.

'Just play ace and another, the contract can't fail. It's an elementary safety play.'

Sir Marcus turned to Philip.

'Looks like the rubber's going to take a little longer than anticipated,' he said drily.

The sharp-eyed lady's eyes narrowed crossly. She snatched up the second pack of cards and cut them aggressively for the dealer. Philip sat down at another table.

'Please, take your time,' he said airily, but no one was paying him any attention.

After a brisk auction Sir Marcus led a card. The young man in jeans put down his hand. The old man in glasses studied it for a moment then put down his own.

'Ruff on the table and draw trumps. Discard my diamonds on the clubs. Give you a spade. Making six.'

'Nor surprised on that lead!' declared the lady decisively.

Sir Marcus's nostrils flared with irritation. Like most bridge players he was rather better at giving than receiving criticism.

'Eight, I think,' said the old man, looking up from his scoresheet and putting down his pencil.

Sir Marcus snapped open his wallet and counted out £160 in new twenties. His partner wrote a cheque.

'Do you want to cut in?' the old man asked, turning to Philip.

Philip came to the table. All five of them drew cards. Philip and Sir Marcus both pulled red aces.

'Can't argue with that,' said the old man, rising from the table. 'Looks like I'm sitting this one out.'

Sir Marcus, who had drawn the ace of hearts, elected to remain where he was. Philip took the seat of the sharp-eyed lady.

'I am Mrs Reizenstein,' she said as she resettled herself opposite her new partner.

'Mal,' said the young man in jeans.

'Dalrymple.'

'Walsingham.'

The introductions over, Mrs Reizenstein cut the pack for Sir Marcus to deal.

'What do you play?'

Philip shrugged.

'I'm easy, old boy. What do you like?'

'Standard Acol. Weak twos, intermediate jumps, Sputnik, u.c.b., Gerber over no trumps, Swiss, Michaels, Stayman, Flint, Backwood. Let's keep it simple. Do you like Fishbind or double?'

Philip, whose knowledge of alien tongues took in only a smattering of German and French, had to pause before replying.

'Er, double.'

'Good. I pass.'

'No bid,' said Mrs Reizenstein.

'Three spades,' said Philip. He may have been only a kitchen bridge player, but he knew a pre-emptive hand when he saw one.

'Double.'

'Pass.'

'No bid.'

The final pass sounded ominous. Mal led the ace of clubs and Sir Marcus put down an unattractive and largely pointless dummy. Philip managed to go three off.

'Should have been only two,' Sir Marcus muttered. Philip tried to work out how, but he had no time. The next hand was dealt quickly and the opponents bid without intervention to a game in no trumps. Mrs Reizenstein made eleven tricks. On the next hand she ended up in a heart slam after her partner had opened a spade.

'Double!' said Sir Marcus with crisp brutality.

Philip stared hard at his hand. It wasn't quite a Yarborough; he had one jack. After a moment's blank reflection he led a top-of-nothing diamond.

Dummy had two singletons, diamonds and hearts. Sir Marcus's diamond king went under Mrs Reizenstein's ace, and she discarded dummy's heart on the queen. She ruffed a heart on the table, drew trumps in two rounds and claimed the contract with an overtrick. Sir Marcus's face had turned white. He addressed Philip with barely controlled fury:

'When your book on opening leads comes out, partner, remind me not to buy a copy.'

'Really?' said Philip innocently. 'Nothing we could have done there, surely?'

Philip's remark made Sir Marcus livid.

'Lead a spade, you bloody fool!'

'I say, old boy, keep your hair on!' said Philip, chuckling amiably.

'That's twenty-seven, I think,' said Mrs Reizenstein.

Sir Marcus took out his wallet, looked at it grimly and put it away again. He reached for his chequebook.

Philip took a thick brown paper envelope out of his inside pocket, opened it and casually shook on to the table five thousand pounds in denominations of twenty and ten. He counted out loud until he'd reached £540 and cheerfully offered the fistful of cash to Mal.

'Don't spend it all at once!' he advised, still chuckling.

He stuffed his remaining cash back into the envelope and returned it to his inside pocket with an unconcerned air, though in reality he was rather shocked. He had been expecting to lose a little, but not this much and certainly not this fast. He had learnt how to play bridge on tour twenty years ago and had been under the impression for most of that time that he was reasonably competent. The sudden realization that he was not had come as a blow.

'At least you don't have to play with me again!' he said to Sir Marcus in a friendly way. The rubber over, all five of them cut again. This time Mrs Reizenstein sat out, and Philip partnered Mal against Sir Marcus and the man with glasses.

'We've not played together before,' said Mal. 'Basic stuff, OK? Weak, Stayman, double.'

'Right.' Philip turned to Sir Marcus. 'Dalrymple – you know, that sounds familiar. We weren't at school together, were we?'

'I shouldn't have thought so. Would you cut, please?'

Sir Marcus dealt and passed. Mal bid a heart and jumped to game after Philip's minimal response. He made an over-trick. Mal dealt the next hand while Philip shuffled.

'Dalrymple, Dalrymple . . .' Philip muttered amiably. 'Does sound awfully familiar.'

'Really?'

'Good God!' said Philip suddenly. 'It's Spanker Dalrymple of the Remove!'

Sir Marcus had just picked up his hand. He slammed it down again on the table.

'What did you say your name was?'

'Walsingham, but call me Frank –'

'No, thank you. I should be grateful, Walsingham, if you would keep your inane witterings to yourself. This is a bridge club, not a social institution. Now can we please bid this hand?'

It didn't take long. This time Mal didn't require any support at all from Philip. He simply opened with a game

161

call and made it on the button. The rubber had taken about two minutes.

'That's that, then!' said Philip, looking with relief at his scorecard. 'I make it ten.'

'Sounds good to me,' said Mal.

It didn't sound so good to Sir Marcus. With the greatest reluctance he removed £200 in cash from his wallet (about all he had left) and tried to pass it to Mal. But Mal was already accepting payment from the man with glasses. With even greater reluctance Sir Marcus gave his money to Philip.

'Cheer up!' said Philip as irritatingly as he could. 'It may never happen.'

'Table up,' said Mal. Two new players had appeared during the rubber. They and Mrs Reizenstein came over to draw a card.

'I think I'll sit out for a while,' said Sir Marcus stiffly. He headed for the door.

'Mm, me too,' said Philip, as soon as Sir Marcus had left the room.

'Are you sure?' asked Mrs Reizenstein. 'You've only just got here.'

'I think so. Thank you for the game.'

Philip caught up with Sir Marcus in the bar downstairs. He literally turned his back on him, picked up the drink he'd just ordered and retired to the farthest corner of the room, where he immured himself behind a copy of the *Spectator*. Philip ordered another drink himself and remained at the bar, biding his time.

After about ten minutes Sir Marcus got up and made for the door. Philip knocked back the remains of his drink and followed him out. Sir Marcus went down to the end of the corridor and into the Gents.

He was at the row of urinals, his back to the door, when Philip walked in. He didn't see him. When he had finished and zipped himself up he turned and made for the washbasins, where Philip was waiting quietly. Sir Marcus did a double-take.

'You know, I'm positive I've seen you somewhere,' said Philip.

Sir Marcus did not reply at once. Methodically he washed and dried his hands, pulling down a length of clean towel with a controlled aggressive tug. He was obviously composing himself. When he was quite ready he turned round slowly, a cold and steely look in his eyes. Philip was impressed. With his natural legal gravitas he'd have been excellent casting for the Inquisitor in *St Joan*.

'I don't know who you are, and I don't know why you are following me about, but if you persist in foisting your unwanted attentions upon me you shall leave me with no option but to call the club manager and have you expelled. I would suggest that you leave quietly now. Excuse me, you're in my way.'

Philip remained where he was, blocking the door. Physical threat was hardly in his armoury, but he could put a sinister glint into his eye when needed. And into his voice. He leant back casually against the door.

'I remember where I've seen you before. Of course. In Bosie Butterflys.'

Sir Marcus didn't bat an eyelid.

'I've no idea what you're talking about. Out of my –'

'Oh, I think you do, Sir Marcus. Or should that be Lady Marcia?'

An eyelid batted; a lip twitched; a tiny droplet of sweat appeared on the forehead.

'Get out of my way, or –'

'Or what?' demanded Philip, his voice a mix of scorn and amusement. Sir Marcus's twitching became more pronounced.

'Who the bloody hell are you?'

'It's not who I am that should concern you. It's what I

represent. You're fishing in dangerous waters, Dalrymple. I'm here to offer a friendly word of warning.'

'Warning about what? I don't have the slightest idea –'

'Oh, I think you do . . .'

From his inside pocket Philip produced the polaroid photograph he'd taken last night. Sir Marcus stared in shock at the picture of him in his carrot wig propped up between Melanie and Rita.

'What are you suggesting? I've never seen these people –'

'Come, come!' Philip laughed richly.

A glimmer of hope appeared in Sir Marcus's desperate eyes.

'Oh, er, I remember now, it was a fancy-dress party –'

'Not bad, not bad – but not quite good enough either. Sorry about this, old man, but your goose is pretty well overcooked. Don't give a damn about the cross-dressing – private life your own affair and all that – but you're mixing with some dodgy characters. We in the Organization have had our eye on Doris Afternoon and cronies for some time now. I must say we were a little surprised to find someone of your eminence cropping up.'

'What Organization?'

'No names, no pack drill. Let's just say we're not the Girl Guides, and we take a pretty dim view of an upright fellow like you compromising national security.'

'National . . . what on earth are you talking about!'

'We've had Bosie Butterflys under electronic surveillance for some time. Late last night we picked up two telephone conversations between you and a Mr Vincent Dorigo. Can you explain their content?'

Sir Marcus's natural presence of mind appeared to have gone absent without leave. The muscles round the eyes flickered continuously, but the pupils themselves were blank. His mouth hung open; the tip of his tongue protruded gormlessly. His voice was dry and cracked.

164

'I . . . I don't . . . what conver . . . Vincent who?'

The last, delivered in a sharply rhetorical manner, seemed to be a final desperate effort to reassert his old authority and rescue himself from catastrophe. It was a futile attempt.

'Vincent Dorigo. Or Colonel Oleg Andropov, as he is better known in certain circles.'

Sir Marcus's lips gave the impression of movement, but no sound came out. Philip permitted himself a look of mild surprise.

'My dear chap, you're not trying to tell me you don't know that Vincent Dorigo isn't his real name? Good God!'

Philip abandoned himself to sardonic laughter. It helped relieve his own tension. Sir Marcus, alas, was beyond relief. He fell back heavily against the nearest washbasin.

'I . . . I don't . . . I know nothing at all!'

'Nothing at all?' Philip repeated softly. 'Come, come, I think you know quite a lot. I think you know that you're up to your neck in something, only perhaps you're not quite sure what it is. That much I'm prepared to grant you, and that's why I'm here, to have a little talk with you before it's too late, before your career, your family life and your position in society are irretrievably damaged. As I'm sure I don't have to tell you, a prison sentence would result in disbarment from your profession, not to mention loss of your title.'

'Prison?' repeated Sir Marcus almost inaudibly.

'Conspiracy to blackmail was against the law last time I checked. We've got the classic ingredients for a great man's fall, and I'm not talking about Nigel Loseby, Sir Marcus. Just think what the newspapers will make of you in this charming little photograph and in cahoots with a renegade KGB officer to boot! Remember the treatment old Blunt got? I certainly do, I was interrogating him at the time!'

'But –'

'But nothing, Sir Marcus. Dorigo – Andropov, I should

165

say – is a rogue element, what we used to call a sleeper in the good old days. Been cooking up his little destabilization wheezes all these years, then bingo! Moscow Central tell him it's all up, forget the Cold War routines, comrade, you'd better pop back home for debriefing. Only five years on the priority housing list, my dear fellow, and in the meantime your pension should just be enough to keep you in cabbage soup. Get the picture? Andropov did, and he didn't like it. Decided to carve out a solo career, make a stash against a rainy day. Perfectly predictable he should try and double-cross Doris and Norman, but frankly we were just a tiny mite surprised that you seem to have fallen for his scam. You don't think for a moment, do you, that he has the slightest intention of cutting you in?'

'But –'

'Excuse me a moment,' interrupted Philip brusquely, putting his hand into his pocket. 'Urgent call.'

The mobile phone he took out of his pocket was a toy he had acquired in a novelty shop. It was a realistic-looking but empty case with all the right buttons and an additional switch which, when pressed, emitted an authentic ringing tone. It was an ingenious device designed to bolster self-esteem in public places, though it could serve its purpose just as well in the privacy of a gentlemen's cloakroom. Philip pressed the button to switch off the tone, then pretended to be listening. His brow furrowed intently.

'Good God!' he exclaimed into the receiver. 'Are you sure about that?'

He counted to five and then, with a grim expression, returned the phone to his pocket.

'I'm very sorry about this,' he said quietly to Sir Marcus, 'but it appears there's been a change of plan. The only advice I can give you is to lie low, though I don't suppose it'll do any good. I'm afraid you're well up shit creek without a paddle. Without a raft, come to that. Best of British, old man.'

166

With a reluctant sigh, Philip turned and walked towards the door. Before he could open it Sir Marcus grabbed him desperately by the arm.

'Where are you going? You can't leave me like this. What's going on?'

He was shaking and on the point of tears. Philip shrugged.

'Can't discuss it any further, I'm afraid, it's classified. I'd forget this conversation has taken place if I were you. Start bracing yourself for the media coverage. Sorry, it's not going to be pleasant –'

'Please!'

It was an animal plea for help. Sir Marcus could contain himself no longer. He sank to his knees, flung his arms round Philip's legs and broke into violent sobs.

'Please! Please! You've got to help me. I know nothing, I'm just a pawn, they're using me, I'll do anything you want, anything, anything, anything!'

'Steady on.'

None too gently Philip pushed Sir Marcus's hands away, grabbed him under the armpits and yanked him to his feet.

'Pull yourself together,' he ordered disapprovingly. 'Stiff upper lip, and all that!'

He didn't have a stiff anything just at the moment; he was like the Michelin man in a heatwave.

'I don't know what Dorigo's up to, I promise. He and Doris just came to me for advice, I told them to get lost but they threatened to expose me if I didn't help. I've got contacts in Fleet Street, they said all they wanted was some introductions, I had no idea what they were planning. I'm not doing it for money, there's nothing in it for me. You've got to believe me!'

Philip pretended to hesitate. He turned away and walked slowly past the washbasins, apparently deep in thought. After a long pause for effect he looked back neutrally at the grovelling wreck by the door.

'All right, I may be able to do something. It's possible, just possible, there's a way to keep your name out of this. I trust that you're going to prove cooperative?'

The look in Sir Marcus's eyes was enough to suggest that on Philip's word he would have dived into boiling oil.

'Good,' said Philip matter-of-factly, with a glance at his watch. He was due at the club in a little over two hours for a rehearsal, which after last night's fiasco he couldn't afford to miss. He also had to pick up another costume from Denis. He took a card out of his breast pocket and handed it over. 'Know this place?'

Sir Marcus read the address on the card and shook his head.

'It's a small hotel, just off the Bayswater Road. Nothing grand. Here.' Philip took from his pocket the key to the room he had booked into as Marlene von Trapp. 'Take this. You're to go straight up to the room and wait. You're not to speak to anyone, anyone at all, and remember – we'll be watching you, every step of the way. Wait by the phone until I call you. Should be in a couple of hours.'

'But tonight I'm due –'

'If you so much as speak to a soul without my express say-so, I'm afraid I shan't answer for the consequences. Understood?'

Sir Marcus's pained silence bore ample testimony to his complete comprehension. Philip took his elbow and pro-pelled him towards the door.

'Remember – we'll be watching you every step of the way.'

Sir Marcus went without another word. As the door swung shut behind him Philip caught a glimpse of himself in the mirror over the basins.

'Jolly good show, Walsingham, old chap. You could lie for England!'

He noticed a gleam of moisture on his forehead. He felt hot under the thick material. He was looking forward

168

to slipping into something more comfortable back at Conchita's flat.

He left the bridge club and headed for Kensington High Street. The first cab he saw was full, and it was heading the other way. Sir Marcus Dalrymple was in the back, white-faced and tight-lipped. Philip suspected that he would take his order of silence literally. He hoped for his sake that the taxi driver wasn't of the garrulous variety.

Philip found a cab of his own a minute later. He sat in the back, sweating into his stiff tweeds and thinking through the various ramifications of his plot. Sir Marcus, as the one with most to lose, had always been the potential weak link. Nevertheless, he'd been lucky the way things had fallen into place. Vincent, Doris and Norman were a different matter altogether. Luck wasn't going to be nearly enough; what was needed was skill and careful planning, not to mention nerves of steel, electric wits and sheer acting perfection.

Just as well he was on the job, really, was his inescapable conclusion.

13

'And now, ladies and gentlemen (and all you in-betweenies), will you give a very special welcome to our star import, back by popular demand, the amazing, the stunning, the marvellous, magnificent, man-eating Marlene, better known as – Miss von Whiplash!'

Philip, behind his curtain, heard and felt the roar of excitement. He waited complacently. The phrase 'by popular demand' was more than mere hype: his dressing room had been inundated with flowers, cards, and discreet invitations. Doris must have been furious. Philip allowed the applause to climb to its peak, and then, just as the wave broke, he threw back the curtain with the arrogant flourish of a matador and strode into the pink arena.

The audience gasped. Philip cracked his whip.

'Ssh! naughty boys, or I vill chastise ze lot of you.'

He flicked the whip again, then stood insolently with his hands on his hips and gave time for the audience to drink him in. He was quite a sight.

Shiny high-heeled jackboots sheathed his calves and hugged his knees. Fishnet stockings, suspended from a wickedly wired corset, caressed his thighs. The matching black SS officer's jacket was left teasingly unbuttoned. A jauntily angled leather cap and swastika armband rounded off the ensemble. The six-foot bullwhip added a final tasteful touch.

'Ach so!' Philip drawled, tapping his toes and eyeing up

the audience shrewdly. 'Vat haf we here? I've never seen such a kinky crew!'

Somebody at the back shouted out something about a pot and a kettle.

'Looks like you're ze first for ze punishment cell,' called back Philip sternly. 'Und zat's with ze emphasis on punishment, sveetie.'

A communal sigh of envy rose from the packed ranks in the pit.

'Don't vorry, darlinks,' said Philip soothingly, 'you'll all get your turn. Starting viz you!'

He lashed out with his whip at the piano. The sound of the leather tip smacking the wood was as loud as a gunshot. Norman jumped up from his stool like a startled rabbit.

'Just play, dummkopf!' Philip snarled at him. 'If you know vat's gut for you . . .'

Norman knew what was good for him. He began to play the opening bars of 'Cabaret', which they had spent the late afternoon rehearsing. Philip transferred his whip to his left hand and picked up the microphone with his right.

It wasn't exactly a conventional Sally Bowles, but nor was Philip exactly a conventional artiste. Throwing himself into the part with gusto, he camped it up to the hilt. A lifetime of rubbing shoulders with the cream of the acting profession had amply prepared him for the task in hand.

The applause that swelled at the dying bars was like the roar in the Colosseum after a jamboree slaughter. The basement air was thick with animal excitement. Philip strutted about the stage like a gladiator, inciting it. The animus of performance inhabited him; he could not help but be intoxicated by his success.

'Ach so . . .' he drawled, singling out a likely-looking customer in the front row. 'How do you like ze show, sveetie – kinky enough for you?'

A thin, nervous voice, barely audible above the hubbub, said that it was very enjoyable, thanks.

'Enjoyable, hah! I think you're getting ze wrong end of the stick. Come and see me afterwards and I'll show you ze right end!'

A heckler safely in the far shadows made an incoherent suggestion.

'Button your lip, schweinhund!' snarled Philip, flicking his whip. 'Or you'll get more zan ze lash of my tongue!'

Out of the corner of his eye Philip noted Norman twitching agitatedly. That didn't bother him (he knew how to handle Norman), but somewhere Doris might be lurking. Tomorrow they could all go to hell; tonight it was make or break. He had better be cautious.

'All right, maestro,' he said to Norman with heavily emphasized irony. 'Let's get on viz it . . .'

Philip settled himself back languidly on the tall barstool behind the microphone stand. A pool of bright white light encircled him. He angled back his leather cap still further and sang Lili Marleen.

The song had a natural haunting quality that not even the limitations of Philip's voice could smother altogether. Though his German was basic he had a good ear. He could act the lyrics, which he'd learnt phonetically, and he could act the part of the singer. He was already acting the part of a man pretending to be a woman – one layer more was neither here nor there. And if anyone in the audience detected a false note in his accent, what did it matter? They were all more or less faking it anyway.

The rowdy audience was moved to silence. Even Norman played with a lightness of touch never hinted at before. The cries of 'Encore!' that greeted the final bars were the most heartfelt yet. Philip was almost sorry to decline.

'Tanks, but no tanks,' he said as he rose from his stool. 'Something to remember me by . . .'

He took off his leather cap and tossed it into the heart of the audience. There was a brief scrabbled frenzy, like a shoal of fish rising for food. Philip backed away towards the curtain, blowing kisses to left and right.

'Auf wiedersehen, sweeties!' he called out, and cracked his whip and left.

The applause continued long after he had left the stage. He heard it in the dressing room, coming through the tannoy. Doris heard it too. He sat silently on the stool facing his bloated made-up face, each clap and cheer draining the colour from his whorish cheeks. He did not speak to or even glance at Philip. And Philip was happy to reciprocate. He stood silently in the corner, waiting for Doris to finish. He noticed that his collection of cards and flowers had been swept unceremoniously off the table and on to the floor.

'Five minutes, Doris,' announced Sandy from the door.

Doris acknowledged him with a nod. He gave his puffy mouth a last and umpteenth coat of lipstick, draped a bright mauve feather boa over his fat bare shoulders, and rose like a Sumo wrestler from his toilette. At the door it seemed as if he had suddenly become aware of Philip's presence. He glared at him coldly.

'Don't ask me why, but Norman seems to be quite taken with you.'

Philip was counting on it.

'Well, I'm not,' continued Doris in a low and spiteful voice. 'After you've collected your pay packet tonight you can piss off. I don't ever want to see you in this club again, no matter what Norman might say. You get the picture?'

'It's been a pleasure working with you, Miss Afternoon,' answered Philip with deliberate coolness.

Doris looked as if he were considering a wounding riposte, but either none came to him or he thought better of it. He exited wearing an air of contemptuous indifference. It fitted him rather better than his ridiculous costume.

When he had gone, Philip sat down on the stool and faced himself in the mirror. His adrenaline level was still high, but he could feel nervousness returning. The onstage performance was one thing; the offstage drama now ripening was something else.

He had got to Sir Marcus Dalrymple just in time. Frank Walsingham's debriefing, over which Philip had presided by telephone in the interval between the rehearsal and the show, had revealed very little room for manoeuvre.

Sir Marcus, as he was keen to reiterate at every opportunity, had simply been a go-between. He had acted for several of the massmarket tabloids in libel actions, and was well known by name and reputation in the newspaper world. An approach from him, Doris had reckoned, carried its own endorsement of good faith. Sir Marcus had thought otherwise, but, as Philip knew already from his tape of their Monday-morning conversation, Doris and Norman had the wherewithal to put the screws on him, and weren't shy of doing so. Sir Marcus had touted the diaries to selected contacts. One editor in particular had been intrigued, but he had wanted to know more. Sir Marcus had been intending to bring his deputy round to the club later tonight. A sum not unadjacent to a hundred thousand pounds had been discussed, the final figure to depend on the actual diary contents, which Sir Marcus had been told to hint contained some explosive entries and named some very interesting names. He had not seen the diary himself.

Nor had Vincent Dorigo. According to Sir Marcus, Dorigo had been a bit-part player, brought in to add a touch of genuine criminal gravitas to proceedings. Someone had been snooping around, Sir Marcus had confided nervously, some old actor chappie friend of Seymour's who needed frightening off. Dorigo had been enrolled to do just that, in return for an undisclosed but no doubt small slice of the proceeds. Too small, in any event, for Dorigo's liking. This, said Sir Marcus, was something he couldn't understand, because Dorigo had only come on board as an afterthought, so how could he have possibly been the cloak-and-dagger puppeteer deftly pulling all the strings?

Frank Walsingham told him not to be naive. Didn't this 'actor chappie friend of Seymour's' sound just a little on the implausible side? He was probably either a stooge or a set-up. Colonel Andropov was a past master of devious subtlety. How else had he persuaded Sir Marcus to collude with him?

It was not a question Sir Marcus showed any keenness to answer. Apparently Doris and Norman weren't the only ones who knew a few unsavoury details about his private life. He swore that he hadn't known what Dorigo was up to, that he'd just agreed to phone him at the beginning and the end of Doris's performance, that he knew nothing, guessed less, and was, in short, an all-round model of abused innocence –

Frank Walsingham had interrupted his stream of desperate self-justification curtly. Innocence and guilt were technical terms with which the Organization were not overly interested. The only question concerned Sir Marcus's continued willingness to cooperate.

On that, Sir Marcus had assured him grovellingly, he could act as if his life depended on it.

'Not my life I'm bothered about,' responded Frank coolly. 'Got a pen handy? Be ready to take down my instructions. I shall conduct this as a military operation. Let's synchronize watches . . .'

Philip sat in the dressing room watching the minute hand crawl around his watch. It was half past eleven, or 23.30 hours, as Frank would have insisted. Frank had always been a stickler for detail.

Philip was too, on and off the stage. He reapplied his mascara and lipstick, and powdered his painted face. He frowned at himself in the brightly lit mirror. What did he look like?

Like nothing on earth. What did he feel like? Ditto. He was a consummate character actor, always had been, character was the essence, but the paradox of his art was

175

to put on a mask only to reveal himself. That was the point of acting as he knew it, the symbiosis between a made-up exterior and the raw innards of instinct and emotion; the relationship honed and perfected by training, experience and a not inconsiderable natural talent; art imitating or perhaps refracting life. Here it was the other way round.

His Marlene was an imitation of an imitation; he was playing the part of a part, and winging it at that, in a gross state of under-rehearsal. He felt as big a phoney as Doris Afternoon.

He frowned at his hybrid image: false hair; false lashes; false face. Not the most alluring bait he could have imagined. Fortunately his own imaginings were not concerned.

'Who's a lucky boy, zen?' he demanded rhetorically, wrapping the length of his whip tightly round the handle and putting it into his handbag. He got up and put on his long camel coat over his kinky costume, buttoning it to the chin. Through the tannoy he could hear Doris begin his rendition of 'I've Got a Lovely Bunch of Coconuts'. He checked his watch. The timing was spot-on. Sir Marcus would be phoning through in five minutes.

Philip put on his floppy shapeless hat, slung his heavy handbag over his shoulder, and left. He went out by the artistes' exit. As he walked into the entrance lobby he heard the applause for the end of Doris's act welling up from below. It did not seem as loud as his own.

'Good night, Miss von Trapp,' said the doorman respectfully. 'Hope to see you again soon.'

Philip smiled regally. He stepped out into a damp, cold London night.

He walked briskly for ten minutes, to warm himself and kill time. His route described a rough elaborate circle. He ended up at the back of the club facing the mews entrance, by the two pay phones.

'Room thirty-eight, please,' he said to the hotel receptionist when at last he answered. The voice he had put on again was bluff and orotund. He waited impatiently to be connected.

'Dalrymple? It's Walsingham. Report in, and keep it succinct.'

'They'll be on their way shortly.'

'Doris and Andropov?'

'Yes.'

'Doris kick up any fuss?'

'Plenty! She wanted to come on her own, wanted to keep Dorigo, I mean Andropov, out of it.'

'What did you say?'

'What you told me to. That Dorigo needed to be watched, he'd asked me to help him snoop around – look, Walsingham, if any of this gets out, if Doris confronts Dorigo, then my life won't be worth –'

'It'd be worth even less, old boy, if snaps of Lady Marcia started appearing all over the place. I take it you're still keen to avoid that?'

'Yes.'

'Sorry, you're speaking very quietly, I can hardly hear you.'

'I said yes!'

'Good. Did Doris want to bring Norman?'

'No. He's holding the fort. That was the expression she –'

'Did he sound suspicious?'

'Er, no. Annoyed, perhaps, but –'

'And the diary?'

'No. I mean, she asked if she should bring it. I said no, like you told me; I've done everything exactly –'

'I'm sure you have. Don't worry, your cooperation will be fully recorded in my final report. What time did Doris say they'd be round?'

'Not before midnight. Said she'd have to get Vincent to pick her up. He wasn't at the club.'

'Good. You've done very well, Dalrymple. Have you made arrangements to leave the country yet?'

'I've booked a flight tomorrow afternoon. I'll have to go home to get my passport –'

'Send a courier. Have you spoken to your wife?'

'You told me I wasn't to ring anyone –'

'Ring her now. Tell her to pack a bag and get your passport ready. Don't tell her where you are.'

'She's not going to like it.'

'Your domestic problems are not my concern. You've had plenty of time to think up a good story. You can phone your office tomorrow, from the airport. Where are you flying, by the way?'

'Er, the Algarve, as you suggested –'

'Excellent choice. It's deserted this time of year. Have a nice holiday. And remember – if you breathe a word to anyone, don't bother coming back to London. Ever.'

Philip cut off the line, but remained in the phone box. It was a good point of vantage. Sir Marcus's voice had been thin and nervous. How had he sounded to Doris? Not too unnatural, obviously, or he wouldn't have bought the story. And he had bought it – that much Philip could confirm for himself now, as he watched Vincent Dorigo's big silver Volvo turning into the street. He averted his face as the headlamps flashed across the kiosk glass, but the dim shape behind the wheel gave no indication that he'd even noticed him. The car drove into the mews. In the distance Philip heard the muffled slam of the door.

The yarn Sir Marcus had spun Doris was plausible enough. The newspaperman didn't want to be seen in the club. It was too public, he preferred to meet on neutral ground. The lowest level of an underground 24-hour car park near Piccadilly was the appointed place. It would be practically empty after midnight.

It was nearly midnight now. Doris was going to be late. So was the newspaperman, but Doris wasn't to know that for sure. Sir Marcus had merely been instructed to warn him of the possibility, to ensure that Doris and Vincent waited patiently underground, with pound signs shimmering behind their eyes to lighten the subterranean gloom. It would be a long wait.

Philip saw a tiny glow expand behind the mews entrance as the car headlamps came on again. The silver Volvo poked its nose out cautiously into the road, with Vincent hunched over the wheel peering to left and right. There was another, ampler figure in the back. Philip caught a flash of shocking pink as the car accelerated smoothly away.

So now they were all out of the way, Doris, Dorigo, Dalrymple. That left only Norman. Philip took another turn around the block, then walked up to the front of the club.

It was after midnight, midweek closing time. A steady stream of customers flowed out of the front door. Philip chose his moment to descend against the current, and, as someone else came out, he took hold of the open door and slipped back in again.

'Oh, it's you,' said the doorman, sounding surprised but respectful. 'You do know we're closing now?'

'I know. I haf forgotten something.'

The doorman nodded and Philip went on down. The customers he passed on the stairs gushed enthusiastically when they recognized him. He heard Norman before he saw him.

'Drink up and fuck off home!'

There was no temptation to linger with Norman around. The club was almost cleared by the time Philip reached the bottom of the stairs, though it was well within the limits of drinking-up time.

'We're closed!' snarled Norman as Philip appeared. And then he realized who it was. 'Oh, it's you . . .'

His face sprouted a leer. Philip did not respond.

'I am owed some money, ja?' he stated with icy hauteur.

'Oh, ja,' said Norman, like an unlikely Sloane. 'I'll give it to you in cash if you hang on a sec. They're doing the

179

till now. Fancy a drink, Marlene, while you're waiting?'

Philip glanced around dispassionately at the empty tables.

'Vat? Here?'

Norman seemed nonplussed.

'Well . . . where else did you have in mind?'

Philip had a mental image of Rita Hayworth giving Glenn Ford her most languorous heavy-lidded look. He had no idea how it would come out, but he tried it on Norman.

'I vas thinking perhaps of somevere a little more . . . intimate.'

He wondered if he were overdoing the fluttering lashes; it might just have looked as if he had grit in his eye. On the other hand, with Norman around subtlety was a complete waste of time.

The leer seemed to freeze on the overstretched face. The eyes glittered momentarily with excitement and calculation. Philip concentrated hard on remaining expressionless.

Norman walked over to the bar. He was trying to appear casual, but there was a dry crack in his voice. He spoke to Sandy at the till.

'Take Miss von Trapp up to the office, will you? Get her a drink. I'll finish off here. You can go home – both of you.'

There was another waiter, washing up behind the bar. He and Sandy exchanged knowing glances. Norman scowled.

'Take her up now, Sandy – not the day after tomorrow.'

Sandy scuttled away quickly.

'This way, Miss von Trapp.'

Philip knew the way perfectly well. Sandy had a key to the office. He ushered Philip in, then went straight to the desk drawer where Doris kept the booze.

'Not much choice, I'm afraid,' commented Sandy.

'I'll haf a Scotch, neat.'

'Oh yeah, we've got Scotch.'

Philip knew that. He could have told him the label. Sandy invited him to sit down.

'If you can find anywhere . . .'

Philip removed some files from a tatty chair and made himself relatively comfortable. Sandy brought him a generous whisky.

'Good night, Miss von Trapp.'

Philip sipped sparingly at his drink. He needed to keep a clear head. He craved a cigarette. Norman entered, carrying a black metal cash-box.

'I'll be down in a sec, Sandy,' he called back over his shoulder. 'All right, Marlene?'

Philip glanced with distaste at his surroundings.

'Ja, I suppose – if you like rubbish dumps.'

'Well, we could go somewhere a little more . . . comfortable.'

'Sounds gut to me, sveetie.'

Philip picked up his drink and followed him out of the office, down the corridor, then to the right. Norman unlocked the bedroom door.

'Much comfier, don't you think?' he breathed suggestively in Philip's ear.

Philip pretended to be looking around for the first time.

'Don't you two ever do any dusting?'

'It's Doris,' said Norman hastily. 'She's a terrible slut. Not like you, Marlene. You're pure class. Have I ever told you that?'

'Nein,' answered Philip with a yawn. 'But plenty of others haf.'

Norman cradled the cash-box under his left arm while he fished in his right trouser pocket.

'Just got to put this away in the safe,' he explained, rattling a bunch of keys. 'I'll have to pop back down to see Sandy out, then I'll be . . . all yours. Won't be a sec. Please make yourself at home.'

Norman scurried away back down the corridor. Philip didn't think he'd be gone long.

He took off his camel coat and bag and hung them on a hook behind the door, which he pushed shut. He took his revolver from the bag, and transferred it to one of his deep jacket pockets. He uncoiled his whip and repositioned himself by the bed. He had brought his drink with him. He took a last quick fortifying slug as he heard Norman's eager squeaking footsteps out in the corridor. A moment later he came crashing through the door.

'Sorry to keep you –'

Philip flicked his whip at Norman's ankles. Norman yelped.

'Vere haf you been, naughty boy? How dare you keep me vaiting!'

Philip stamped his jackboot angrily on the floor. He took a menacing step towards Norman.

'Zese boots vere made for valking, schweinhund. Und zey're going to valk all over you if you don't start behaving yourself!'

Another crack of the whip had Norman cowering in the corner.

'Please, please don't hit me!' Norman begged, sounding suspiciously as if he meant the opposite.

'Take off your trousers!'

Norman tripped over himself in his eagerness to get them off. A packet of cigarettes fell out of one of the pockets, then some coins, then some matches, then a bunch of keys. The biggest of them, heavy and black, gleamed dully on the carpet.

'Bend over!'

Norman bounced over to the bed on his knees, his arms thrust forward and hands clasped together in a gesture of perverted supplication.

'Don't hit me, please, please! I promise I won't be a naughty boy again!'

'Too late!' snarled Philip sadistically. 'You need to be taught a lesson. Zere is no one left downstairs, ja?'

'They've all gone home –'

'Gut. Zen zere vill be no one to hear you scream . . .'

Philip stood astride Norman's thin white legs, smacking the whip handle into his palm.

'I'm pleased to say zis is going to really hurt, baby . . .'

Norman gave an expectant whimper.

'Zere's only one thing to do viz naughty boys like you. Close your eyes!'

Philip dropped the whip on to the bed and grabbed Norman by the collar. He took the revolver out of his pocket, grasping it by the stubby barrel.

'Auf wiedersehen, sveetie!'

He brought the butt of the gun down hard on the base of the balding skull. Norman slumped forward noiselessly.

He didn't appear to be breathing. For a moment Philip wondered if he'd killed him, but he always wondered that after coshing someone, it was force of habit. He bent down, lifted up an eyelid and saw the eye flicker. It would take more than one blow to the head to dispose of leathery old Norman.

Philip climbed up on to the bed, grabbed the inert body under the armpits and dragged it up. He found the leather thongs attached to the bed legs and tied Norman's wrists and ankles securely. In other circumstances Norman would surely have been thrilled.

Philip picked up the bunch of keys and strode rapidly down to the office. The glass door was locked. He found the right key, opened it and marched straight over to the empty filing cabinet in the corner. He flung it aside.

The big black key fitted smoothly into the safe lock. He turned it and heard a heavy satisfying clunk. He depressed the lever and pulled open the door.

Beyond the door was a shallow cavity, beyond that a

183

bare brick wall. A second safe was set in the wall. He tried the handle.

It wouldn't budge. There was no point looking at the bunch of keys. It was a combination lock. He couldn't believe his rotten luck. He threw down the keys in disgust.

He returned to the bedroom. Norman was still unconscious. He slapped his cheek, got no response. He went next door to the bathroom, threw the toothbrushes out of their mug and filled it with cold water.

Norman twitched as the water drenched his face. After a second a low moan escaped his lips. Philip knelt astride him and shook his shoulders until he came round.

'I haf some questions to ask you, Britischer pig-dog,' said Philip, like a uniquely camp commandant. He'd never again be able to view *The Colditz Story* in the same light. He moved to the side of the bed. A single bloodshot eye stared back at him unsteadily.

'What?'

The eye was blank, uncomprehending. Now was the time to strike, before full consciousness returned, while the fuzzily aware portion of Norman's brain might still mistake the interrogation for a game.

'Ve haf ways of making you talk,' said Philip with menace, bending over him and offering his coiled whip for inspection. He said suddenly: 'What is the combination of the safe in the office?'

The stare remained blank. Philip gave Norman an impatient nudge.

'Ze combination! Schnell!'

Norman's brow contracted. A glimmer of understanding came into his eye.

'You bitch!'

Philip raised an eyebrow.

'Zat's no vay to talk to a lady.'

Norman called him something colourfully Teutonic in round Anglo-Saxon.

'I vill give you one last chance!' announced Philip angrily, tautening a length of whip between his fists. 'Ze combination – or else!'

Norman said nothing. He just spat into the pillow.

'You asked for it, sveetie. Und I tell you, zis is going to hurt you a great deal more zan it's going to hurt me . . .'

For the next five minutes Philip flogged Norman mercilessly. At least he still had on his shirt to cover his back, but thick red weals soon sprang up all over his naked legs and buttocks. His pitiful yelps might have given a lesser-hearted man pause, but Philip had a job to do and he stuck to it manfully.

'Had enough?' he demanded, when he judged he had made his point. 'Ze combination!'

'Go to hell!'

Philip's arm was aching furiously. He stopped for a moment to take a sip of his drink. Norman, spreadeagled and restricted as he was, had craned his neck around sufficiently to get a look at him. There was a mocking glint in his eye.

'That the hardest you can hit, then?'

It occurred to Philip that torturing a masochist was a contradiction in terms. He might just as well have been flogging a dead horse.

Calmly he took the gun out of his pocket and pressed the tip of the barrel into Norman's face.

'Ze combination, or I redistribute your stinking brain cells over ze pillow.'

Norman laughed hoarsely.

'Then you'll never know it, will you?'

Reluctantly Philip was forced to concede the point. Alas, Norman was no coward. Years of vigorous punishment had hardened him. A more drastic solution was required.

'Don't go away,' murmured Philip, putting away his gun after a long moment's thought.

He marched out of the bedroom, back along the corridor,

past the office. He fumbled for the right light switches, then went down the stairs to the first landing.

The ring of a telephone startled him. It was faint and far behind him, probably coming from the bedroom. It didn't matter, Norman was in no position to answer. If it were Doris calling, he might be suspicious. Who else could it be but Doris, at this time of night? Philip quickened his step.

The key to the garage was on the hook where it should have been. Everything in the garage was exactly as he remembered it. The can of petrol was on the floor by the outer door.

The can was heavy, at least half full. The liquid sloshed around noisily as he carried it back up the stairs. The phone was no longer ringing.

The mockery was still there in Norman's expression. Philip didn't expect it to remain in place long. He unscrewed the cap as he carried the can over to the bed.

'What you doing?'

Philip said nothing. Silence was more threatening. He began to pour the petrol over Norman.

'Hey! That hurts!'

Philip wasn't surprised. The legs were red and raw. He started at the feet, and poured upwards, taking his time to drench the shirt. There was plenty in the can. He emptied a last generous measure over Norman's head.

He picked up the box of matches from the floor and struck one.

'Hey!'

He flicked the match at the petrol-soaked body. It went out in the air immediately, but from Norman's screams one might have judged otherwise. Philip lit another match, and held it up between finger and thumb.

'The combination?'

'Twelve-eleven-forty-six – Doris's birthday!'

Nine times out of ten it was something ridiculously simple like that. Philip blew out the match.

'Do be quiet!' he muttered.

Norman was shaking and sobbing. Philip stepped back. Either the noise or the petrol fumes was addling his brains. He'd forgotten the numbers already.

'What was the combination again?'

'Twelve-eleven-forty-six,' said a voice behind him. 'My birthday.'

As he turned around Philip caught a glimpse of Doris's shape in the door. It was the last thing he did glimpse for some little time.

Something that felt like a ton of cement had just smashed into the side of his head.

14

He wasn't aware of anything except pain. Consciousness
flickered on and off. He was dimly aware of discomfort at
being pulled about, handled roughly, but it was nothing
to the ache in his head.

He heard voices. He had no idea to whom they belonged,
whether or not they were even real: he heard sounds, not
words; they could just have been buzzing inside his skull.
The voices dripped into his head, like the water torture.
He could have screamed, had he remembered how it was
done.

One time he came round the pain was a little less, a
dull flat hammering on the nerves, not the usual insistent
violent assault with a pickaxe. Those Chinese whispers
were still volleying back and forth between his ears. Buzz,
buzz, they went. A hint of sense formed somewhere in the
bruised chaos of his brain, despite the lapping waves of
pain.

'It hurts!' whined a voice that was wounded but wasn't
his own.

'Of course it hurts, you big pansy,' came the less than
sympathetic reply. 'It's the petrol in your cuts. Serves you
right, what have I always told you about S&M and
strangers?'

'I'll kill the fucking bitch!'

And then he was being hit – kicked or punched, he
couldn't tell, it didn't matter, the blows were hard and

excruciating and crushed what little sense had crept back into his skull. The agony was unbearable. His brain blotted it out and slipped back into oblivion.

Some other time, and he was hearing voices again, one moment far away, the next seemingly loud in his ear. They might have been real, or they might have been part of his dream. His veiled consciousness was awash with images and noise. It was a terrible dream.

People were trying to hurt him. He couldn't see their faces, but he could feel their hatred, their cruel intent. Why me? he asked them in his dream, why do you want to harm me, lovable little me, who's never hurt a fly? The masked faces laughed satirically. Your just deserts at last, said a dry mocking voice that sounded, as they all did, unpleasantly familiar. He had the uncomfortable conviction that he'd done a lot of people wrong. The faces were grinning still. There'll be laughter in hell tonight, said one, and they all laughed louder. Where I am is hell, he thought mechanically, and another voice told him with relish that he'd better believe it. Why were there so many who didn't like him? How had he undone so many? Was there no end to this queue of phantoms? How could he know what he'd done? He didn't even know who he was. A shrill, irritating ringing noise interrupted the raucous voices. Ringing out the old –

'Don't expect sympathy from us!' A female ghost was singing in his ear. 'You self-centred egotistical bastard, Philip Fletcher!'

He gasped. A cold chill shot through his system, an icy implosion of terror and remorse. The throbbing pain hadn't gone away, but somehow it had been pushed to the side. Everything was submerged in fear.

He knew who he was now, and once he knew that he understood where he was, and that he was in terrible danger. He was lying on the bed, and he couldn't move. His feet were tied together, and so were his hands, behind his back. The voices he heard were not inside his head.

'It's Vincent,' said Doris Afternoon. The jarring ringing noise had stopped. It had been the telephone. Philip heard the distorted electronic murmur of Vincent Dorigo's voice.

'It's as I thought, Marcus has scarpered,' reported Doris, and then, into the phone: 'Yeah. See you soon.'

'I'll kill the bastard,' said Norman savagely. 'After I've finished with this heap of shit.'

A heavy boot struck Philip a glancing blow on the leg. His body was so numb already he hardly felt it, but in any case, he didn't dare react: trussed and helpless as he was, the only advantage that he had was that they still thought him unconscious. He kept his eyes tight shut, and metaphorically bit his lip.

'Marcus's wife says she hasn't a clue where he is.'

'Did Vince believe her?'

'Yeah. Said she was hopping mad with him. She was still up waiting, hadn't gone to bed. He was supposed to take her to some do tonight, give a speech, just didn't turn up, not a word of explanation, left everyone in the lurch. Then about an hour ago he rings up, asks her to pack a few clothes and his passport for him, says he's got to leave the country suddenly.'

'The only place he's going is in a wooden box.'

'My thoughts exactly. The wife's gone ballistic, told him to go screw himself, said it was good for him he was a solicitor, he could handle his own divorce.'

'Someone should tell her widows don't need a divorce.'

'I know that, and you know that, Norman. And Vincent knows it, but he's got enough brains not to let Lady Dalrymple in on it too.'

'I was just saying –'

'You don't have to, just shut it!'

'Don't get ratty with me, I'm the one who's suffered –'

'You bloody would have suffered if you'd lost that diary,

190

I'm telling you. What did you give her the combination for?'

'What choice did I have? I only thought she was after the cash –'

'How bloody naive can you get! Marked down as a sucker from the start, you were. Good thing for you I've got better than grade-A sawdust packed between my ears. If you'd been in my place you'd still be sitting in that stupid car park.'

'I've said how grateful I am.'

'I smelt a rat from the off. You're lucky I've got a good nose. Marcus sounded weird on the phone, I knew something was up. I wasn't going to sit in that car all night, I couldn't have – you should have smelt the garlic on Vincent's breath. That was when I used the carphone, gave Marcus's name at the switchboard and asked how I could get hold of the journalist. I can't say I was a hundred per cent surprised when the night desk told me he was on holiday and wasn't even in London.'

'You're clever, Doris.'

'I am. It was a hunch. You get hunches when you're clever, Norman, I don't suppose you'd know.'

'All right, stop rubbing it in.'

'You'll be lucky. Only question is, where's Marcus now? And is it just these two, or are there more of them in it?'

'That's two questions.'

'Don't get smart with me, Norman. Smart's not your scene.'

'Lay off.'

'I will when you shut your face.'

'Easy enough to find out how many of them are in it.'

'Really? Go on, Norman, amaze me.'

'Get this slag on the bed to talk. Give her the treatment she gave me, I'll have her singing like a bird.'

'All in good time, Norman. We'll wait till Vincent gets back. He's the expert.'

'Don't need an expert. Leave it to me.'

'I'll leave it to all of us together, if you don't mind. What's the point of having Vincent on board if we don't use him? And to think I almost believed that bullshit Marcus was giving me about Vince trying to screw us.'

'Vince is a mate, he wouldn't do that.'

'He's more than a mate, Norman, he's a pro. Worth his weight in gold, and that's why I'm going to wait. He's the one who'll be disposing of the bodies, that's his line. Won't be long till he's here now. Let him earn his money.'

'He's not going to settle for ten per cent now, is he? I'll finish this one off for free, my pleasure, bullet in the – '

'I said we'll leave it to the expert, all right? If we have to up the ante, that's just too bad, it's your fault and no one else's. You don't have a clue; if I let you handle it you'd only screw up again – '

'Shut up!'

'I should have left you tied up on the bed, would have taught you a lesson. Change that shirt, it stinks.'

'It's the petrol.'

'I didn't think it was your aftershave.'

'I haven't got any clean shirts. That's your fault, you slut, you said you'd send the stuff down the laundry – '

'Don't talk to me like that. I've more important things to worry about than your wardrobe.'

'Hark at her!'

'That shirt's damp. You'll catch pneumonia.'

'It's almost dry.'

'Don't blame me if I light a fag and you blow up.'

'How many times have I told you, I don't like you smoking in the bedroom.'

'Don't fucking lecture me!'

'Fuck the fuck off!'

'Ssh! Was that a car?'

'Didn't hear a thing.'

192

'Cloth ears. I think it was. It'll be Vincent. I'll go and check. Don't do a thing till I get back.'

Domestic hostilities temporarily suspended, Philip heard the heavy tread of Doris's footsteps receding down the landing. Norman must have gone into the bathroom, whence came the sound of running water.

Philip opened the corner of one eye. His vision was blurred. He could feel the thick swellings throbbing around his brows; he had a pair of shiners coming on. It made no difference. There was nothing to see. He tried to move. His ankles were bound very tight, pinioned against each other so hard it hurt. He tried his wrists. They were a little better, not loose, but not so tight either as to cut off his circulation. His feet were numb – at least there was feeling in his fingers. His wrists had been bound separately, were linked by an inch or two of what felt like pyjama cord. It didn't leave him much leeway, the knots were tight and Boy Scout thorough. He'd never have been able to pick them out, even had he been able to get at them properly.

He shut his eyes as he heard Norman come back into the bedroom. He must have been standing quite close, he could smell the petrol. He heard the voices of Doris and Vincent coming down the corridor. The tail end of their conversation did nothing to soothe his nerves.

'I've got a gun in the safe, if you need it,' said Doris.

'I always use my own,' answered Vincent softly. 'By the way, the old deal doesn't apply from here on in. If I'm going to do your dirty work I'm looking for a straight three-way split.'

'You've got it.'

Philip's headache hadn't gone, but somehow it was no longer bothering him. Frantically he considered his options. It didn't take long. He didn't have any.

'Wake him up,' Vincent commanded.

Norman grabbed his shoulders and began to shake him.

'Wakey, wakey, you two-timing bitch!'

193

Philip emitted a low moan as he pretended to come round. Norman slapped him repeatedly on the cheek. Philip fluttered his eyelids.

'Ugh . . .' he groaned with conviction. 'Where am I?'

'Never-never land,' said Norman, administering a last gratuitous slap.

'That'll do,' said Vincent.

He had pulled up a chair. He turned it around, sat astride it, and crossed his arms on the tall back. The usual fake puffy pleasantry had fled from his eyes; they had no expression at all. The voice was suitably deadpan.

'I'm going to ask you a few simple questions, all right? I want straight answers. Piss me around, and I'll let Norman sort you out. OK, Norm?'

'OK, Vince,' came the answer in an ominous lip-smacking tone.

Philip couldn't see Norman, but he could hear him pacing about on the other side of the bed. He also heard the sound of him hitting something into his palm.

'Who are you?' asked Vincent.

Philip rolled his eyes groggily.

'I am . . . Marlene,' he said in a slurred voice.

Vincent aimed a tiny signalling glance over his shoulder. The next moment a terrible searing pain ran through Philip's legs. His eyes misted with tears.

'Nasty-looking whip you've got there, Norm,' said Vincent casually, taking out a cigarette and lighting a match. 'Let him have another taste of it.'

'My name's Richard Jones,' blurted out Philip quickly.

He wasn't quite quick enough, because Norman hit him again. But he'd have probably hit him anyway.

'Richard Jones?' said Doris, who was standing behind Vincent. 'Like the actor?'

'Lying bitch!' snarled Norman, and whipped him again.

Philip had never had a high pain threshold, and it had already been uncomfortably exceeded. The whip had been striking him on the bare flesh of his upper thighs, between his corset and stocking tops. The pain was excruciating.

'Hang on,' Vincent murmured thoughtfully. He leant forward, reached for Philip's head and yanked off his blonde wig.

'What you doing?' Doris wanted to know.

'Checking him out,' said Vincent, with a trace of smugness. He stared hard into Philip's face. 'He's an actor, all right, but not the one he just said. It's the bloke you sent me to sort out.'

'What?'

'Look at him. May have more paint on than the Forth bridge, but that's him all right. You're into this crossdressing lark in a big way, aren't you, Mr Fletcher?'

Philip winced inwardly as Norman and Doris drew close to get a better look and three nakedly malicious pairs of eyes raked him over.

'Nice one, Vince,' murmured Doris approvingly. 'Who'd have guessed it, eh?'

'Not me,' muttered a slack-jawed Norman.

'That goes without saying.'

'Piss off!'

'Shut it, you two,' ordered Vincent sternly. 'Leave your bickering till later. I've got some more questions to put to Mr Fletcher.'

Doris and Norman stepped back out of the frame with ill grace. Vincent edged his chair a little nearer. Philip was trembling all over. He realized, somewhat too late, that he had severely underestimated Mr Dorigo.

'Right, Mr Fletcher. Now, who are you working for?'

'No one. I'm unemployed.'

Vincent raised his eyebrow at Norman and the whip came stinging down.

'There's no point in lying, Fletcher,' contributed Doris from the position he had resumed against the wall. 'We know you're working for Seymour's lad.'

'Why would I be doing that?' responded Philip, sounding as composed as he could in the circumstances.

'What do you mean?' demanded Vincent.

'Why should I be working for Nigel?' Philip insisted. 'That diary's a gold mine. I'm working for myself. There are more people than Nigel Loseby would pay to keep it under wraps –'

'How do you know that?' butted in Doris.

'I'm just guessing – but I knew Seymour.'

'Where's Dalrymple?'

'I don't know.'

The beating this time was prolonged and savage. Vincent sat quietly watching while Philip squirmed uselessly.

'All right, Norman,' said Vincent eventually. 'That'll do.'

Norman administered one last lash and then retired. Philip's legs felt as if they had been rolled in a particularly vicious bed of stinging nettles.

'Hurts, doesn't it?' said Vincent with mock-cheerfulness. 'Norman will carry on all night, if I ask him to.'

'Too right!' assented Norman vigorously.

Philip didn't doubt it. But he didn't doubt either that the moment they had extracted all the information they wanted they would have no further use for him, and once that happened his prospects would be distinctly slim.

'Look,' he said, gritting his teeth, 'do you think I wouldn't turn Dalrymple in if I knew where he was? I don't give a damn about him, you can have his balls for breakfast for all I care –'

'We will,' murmured Doris.

'– but the simple fact is that he's done a bunk, and I'm as much in the dark as you are.'

'You and him set this up together, though?' asked Vincent.

'I worked on him the same way you did, threatened to expose him if he didn't cooperate. He's scared shitless, in fact. He said if he didn't hear from me tonight he'd go to the police.'

'Oh really?' said Vincent sarcastically. 'Scared to death of any of this leaking out and you reckon he'll blab to the filth? Didn't nobody ever tell you lying's bad for your health?'

Philip felt almost delirious with shock and hurt. He had to try and get a grip of himself, he couldn't take any more, if Norman so much as threatened him again he might blurt it all out, anything to make him stop. Once he'd done that they would kill him.

That thought cauterized his delirium. It came into his head with sudden singeing clarity, and it lodged there.

They were going to kill him.

It hadn't been meant to turn out like this. Somewhere along the way his carefully crafted plot had been derailed. He'd known what sort of people he was dealing with, Vincent's visit to his flat had been a deliberate warning which he'd ignored. Why hadn't he been more careful? Why hadn't he been quicker? A dash more brio and he'd have been well out of there with the diary stashed safely away. Wisdom after the event was emptying itself over him by the bucketload.

The diary. That was what it all came down to, Seymour's trivial boasts and jots. Hardly a cause worth dying for. Jealousy and greed and vanity and vaulting ambition had undone him. If he did manage to get out of this alive, he thought to himself pitifully, he would resolve to lead a better life.

Doris and Vincent were conversing in whispers. He couldn't make out the words but he didn't like the tone.

'Look,' said Philip quickly. 'I'll do a deal. I've got money, cash. I'll get it for you tomorrow, fifty thousand if you let me go.'

'Oh yeah?' said Doris scornfully. 'Then how come you said you could only go to twenty before?'

'That was Nigel,' said Philip desperately. 'I'm acting for myself now. Sixty thousand – it's all I've got!'

'Bit late for making deals now,' said Vincent coldly. 'I've had enough of listening to this shit. One of you shut him up.'

Doris opened a drawer of the bedside table and took out a roll of brown sticking tape.

'Anything happens to me Marcus is bound to go to the police!'

'And how's he going to know anything's happened to you?' asked Vincent, lighting another cigarette. 'You're about to disappear off the face of this planet . . .'

Norman yanked his head up and held him tightly round the throat while Doris taped up his mouth, unravelling the roll half a dozen times around his head until the gag was tight. Philip could hardly breathe. He was so terrified he hardly even dared breathe, anyway – were they going to do it now?

'You'd better undo his legs,' said Vincent. 'We'll never be able to carry him downstairs.'

Doris and Norman between them untied the knot. Norman grabbed him by the collar and yanked him up into a sitting position. He was pointing Philip's own gun at him.

'Get up!'

So they weren't going to shoot him there and then. It wasn't much to be thankful for. His legs were so weak and bloodless he could hardly stand. He was fighting for breath, his head swam for lack of oxygen. Norman shoved him down the corridor, the barrel of the gun pressed into the small of his back. He heard Vincent's voice behind him.

'It's all right, Doris, you stay here. I'll have Norm to give me a hand. I think he's looking forward to it . . .'

Philip stumbled and almost fell as they reached the top of the stairs. Vincent and Norman held him up between them and half lifted him down to the first landing.

'We'd better make damn sure we get hold of Marcus

after this,' said Norman, as they pulled Philip along to the garage.

'Don't worry about it.'

'But how are we going to find him?'

'No problem. He told his wife he's sending a courier round to his home tomorrow morning for his passport. It doesn't have to be the same courier who turns up at the other end, does it?'

'But . . . oh, I get it!'

They pushed Philip into the garage. Norman unlocked the outer door.

'Wait here while I check it out,' Vincent told him as he went out.

A car engine came on outside. The noise drew closer. Vincent reappeared in the doorway.

'All right, get him out – sharpish!'

Norman shoved Philip through the door with the gun jammed into his back. The mews was empty and deserted. Immediately in front of the garage stood Vincent's car. The boot was open. The light had not been fixed.

Philip tried to struggle but he was too weak. They seized him by the arms, bundled him into the boot and slammed shut the lid.

He lay in the confined darkness, his knees squashed up into his stomach, struggling for breath and listening to the bloody drumbeat pounding through his inner ear. His pulse was in overdrive, sweat and fear poured off him. He pulled with desperate futility at the rope that bound his wrists.

The boot lid was flung up again suddenly. A shape hovered unfocused against the night sky. Was this it, then? He shut his eyes.

Something long and hard was thrown in on top of him. A piece of metal scraped against the side of his head. The boot lid was closed again.

The floor vibrated as the engine revved up. The car began to move.

He felt sick. He swallowed bile, tried to concentrate on breathing regularly. It wasn't easy in his close, black cell. The car stopped suddenly, jerking him backwards. Hard metal pressed into his face again.

It was a spade. He could feel the length of the handle against his body, feel the edge of the blade against his cheek. Why had they packed a spade? Somehow he didn't think they were off on a nocturnal dig for potatoes. He had an awful feeling that Vincent Dorigo had done this sort of thing before. He remembered his little speech about the dangers of finding oneself lying face down in a deserted quarry. It had an uncomfortable ring of experience.

A terrible listlessness had taken hold of him. He was so utterly helpless, there was nothing he could do. Only a miracle could save him, and he didn't believe in miracles.

Vivid images splashed across his brain: he saw the car driving down some beaten track, dense desolate woodland masking the ghastly scene from innocent eyes. At the edge of the quarry they stopped, dragged him from the boot and made him kneel on the cold earth. The barrel of the gun touched the back of his head, and then his life was turned off like a light switch. But the nightmare didn't end there.

Perhaps they would make him dig his own grave first. How long would he lie in it undetected? How long before some stray rambler reported the new suspicious mound? Didn't that always happen, sooner or later?

> But keep the Wolf far thence that's foe to men
> For with his nails he'll dig them up again.

He could see the headlines in the papers. Shock and amazement that ran around the world. The body of the famous actor Philip Fletcher, missing for so many months or years, discovered yesterday in an unmarked grave, badly decomposed but still clearly dressed in women's underwear and a Nazi uniform. Mass suicides reported amongst the members of his thriving and largely female post-humous fan club.

I have lost my reputation. I have lost the
immortal part of myself, and what remains is
bestial . . .

That it should come to this. Woe, alas, and thrice woe! He should volunteer to help dig the grave whether they wanted him to or not. It had better be deep.

He screamed into his gag of tape. Never mind the bullet, he was going to suffocate if this journey lasted much longer. How long had they been driving? He couldn't tell. In his dark cramped prison seconds and minutes had no meaning. All that mattered was the fetid breath he could snatch in through his nostrils, the rapid-fire heartbeat that told him he was still alive. That spark of life was too precious to let go of lightly. He could not give in.

His wrists were red and sore already, but he pulled at the rope with all his strength. It was hopeless, but what else was there to do? The car jolted over a bump and the spade squashed painfully into his nose. The blade was sharp, he could feel it creasing his skin.

He lifted his mouth to the blade, felt it press between his taped lips. It was rounded at the bottom, but right-angled at the top. He craned his neck to get into position, then pecked at the sharp corner like a bird at a milk bottle top.

He punctured the sticky brown tape. The blade scraped against his teeth, he tasted metal. He moved his head from side to side, worked on the hole. He stretched his aching jaws wide and gasped in oxygen.

He took deep lungfuls of the stale air and thought it sweet. It may have been a minor victory, but it was something at least to set against the catalogue of defeats. He had only to imagine the embarrassed tone of his obituary to spur himself on. He thought of Richard Jones devouring

201

the newspaper reports and laughing into his morning cornflakes. Smug Sir Richard Jones.

He pulled in his knees and with an almighty effort rolled himself over. His chin was now up against a tyre. His toes brushed against something metal and square. He remembered that there had been a tool box in the boot that time he had inspected the car. There might be something useful inside, but he couldn't think of a way to get at it. Anyway, he had another idea.

He stretched out his fingertips behind his back and felt for the handle of the spade. He managed to insert the top between his ankles, then pulled it down until the blade was level with his wrists. He used his feet to try and hold it steady, as he worked the rope up and down the sharp edge.

He was so cramped and his position was so awkward that he could bring little pressure to bear. He tried to ignore the ache in his arms, the numb tingling in his blood-starved fingers, and carried on anyway. He had nothing better to do. Up and down he worked the rope, methodically, slowly, trying to hit the same spot over and over. Each time he slackened he thought of his enemy and managed another spurt.

He had to rest though, eventually. Every drop of power had been squeezed from his muscles. With his mouth stretched wide he lay panting for breath. It was fortunate he had never suffered from claustrophobia.

Time dragged on in its meaningless way. How much longer did he have, how many hours or minutes of life? Soon he'd be able to rest for eternity.

He forced himself to start rubbing at his wrists again, but it wasn't doing any good. The spade may have been sharp enough to cut through tape, but the rope seemed scarcely frayed. He could carry on like this for days and not get anywhere. He didn't have days.

He felt for the tool box with his feet, and pulled it along

towards him. It was heavy and full, there had to be something he could use inside. But how could he get at it? He turned himself over again, contorted and twisted until he could feel the outline of the box with his fingers. He tried to tip it over, to get at the lid. He couldn't exert any leverage. Using his feet as well as he could he worked the box along the floor until it was level with his chest. Then he turned himself around once more to face it.

He ran his face along the box, traced its shape with his mouth. He tried to lift the lid with his lip, but it held fast. There was a catch. He remembered now. He licked along the box until he had found it, and attempted to dislodge it with his teeth.

He couldn't get a grip. He kept at it until his neck muscles could take the strain no longer. His head flopped back and smacked into the floor.

His cheek hit something hard and uncomfortable. Hardly a major new grievance to add to his list of woes, but it brought tears of frustration to his eyes. He swivelled his head and flipped the offending object away. It was small and cylindrical.

Small and cylindrical. It jarred his memory. He slid his head across the floor until he was in contact with it again. He ran his tongue along it, recognized the plastic tube, the serrated metal wheel at the top. It was Vincent Dorigo's disposable lighter. He must have dropped it when the policeman had startled him.

In his eagerness to get at it he somehow pushed it further away. He wasted precious moments in retrieving it with his mouth. He lifted his head, flipped the lighter over his body and heard it hit the metal of the spade. This time his fingers closed around it.

He felt for the flame adjuster. It was just as he had left it, on maximum. He pushed his arms as far away from his body as he could and flicked it on. A ruddy glow illuminated the boot interior.

He sat up. He could just manage it if he kept his head fully hunched down. His shoulders, pressed hard into the boot lid, kept him steady. The car seemed to be moving more slowly.

He sat very still, very quietly. At the beginning of the journey he had heard the noise of other cars, but then they had been going faster and he had heard nothing. Now they appeared to be crawling along, but there were no other cars. They passed briefly over something metal and the whole vehicle shook. After that they were driving even more slowly, and the road was very uneven.

The metal had been a cattle grid. The bumpy road meant they were far from London. They were near the spot where they intended to kill him.

The car stopped. He heard a door opening and closing. Long moments passed, then the car started moving again.

Frantically he positioned the lighter under the slack inch or two of rope between his hands and flicked it on. His grip was awkward, he could only guess the angle at which to aim it. He felt something burning. Was it the rope or was it his jacket? He howled with silent anguish as the soft underside of his wrist was scorched. The lighter slipped out of his fingers and he fell back on to his side.

The car stopped again. He lay once more in darkness, filled with dread. He heard the doors slamming, faint voices in the quiet night outside. He closed his eyes.

The boot lid was flung open suddenly and a torch shone in. He turned his face into the floor, hoped they wouldn't see the torn gag. What did it matter? It was all up with him now.

'Got it,' he heard Norman mutter under his breath. The spade was yanked out from under his body. The boot was slammed shut again.

Hardly a reprieve, but a stay of execution at least. They hadn't bothered to scrutinize him; as far as they were concerned he was finished already. In their complacency might lie his salvation.

He sat up again, felt for the right spot in the rope with his fingertips. It was warm. He hadn't just been hurting himself. He flicked the lighter on again.

He could smell the burning rope. Then, suddenly, he could feel it burning his flesh again, and he had to throw his body back on to his wrists to smother the flame. This time the rope was too hot to touch. He got back his breath, summoned up his will, and tried again.

The pattern repeated itself. The rope would smoulder, catch, burn, but then almost at once it would scorch his abused and tender skin and the pain was simply unbearable. He couldn't tell if he was getting anywhere. The gaps between his attempts were growing longer. He could not go on torturing himself forever. He summoned his failing courage one last time, and tried again.

He heard muffled voices outside. They sounded as if they were arguing.

'I want my bit of fun first,' said Norman insistently.

Philip lay back on the floor, clutching the lighter tightly in his fist. It was all he had. He forced himself to ignore the soreness of his skin as he pulled with all his strength at his bindings. Was it his imagination, or was there some give at last?

The boot lid swung up smoothly. Philip averted his gaze from the torch.

'Take his legs,' ordered Vincent.

Norman grabbed him by the ankles and pulled them over the rim of the boot. They each took a lapel and yanked him up and out. He stumbled as his feet hit the ground. He fell into a muddy puddle.

It was a crisp clear night. The silver near-full disc of the moon glowed through the leaves of the tall trees all around him. The car was parked in a narrow path flanked by dense dark woods.

Vincent and Norman dragged him to his feet. Although the night was cold they were both stripped to their shirt-sleeves; they'd been busy, he could smell the sweat on them. No doubt they could smell his, too, his pungent fear.

They frogmarched him off to the left. The undergrowth was soft and spongy. It broke his fall when they threw him down, some twenty yards in from the path.

They were in a tiny clearing. The bright moonlight scarcely penetrated, but Vincent carefully set down his torch on the stump of a tree. It was pointing at a freshly dug hole in the ground. The spade was standing in the loose pile of earth next to it.

'Get him over there,' said Vincent, bending down to the torchlight to see better what he was doing.

He was fitting a silencer to an automatic pistol.

'I said I want my fun first!' said Norman sulkily.

'We haven't got time!'

'We have. Five minutes. After what's been done to me you can spare five minutes.'

'I'm not going to hang around like a lemon while you do your pervy thing!'

'You don't have to watch!'

Vincent muttered something crossly under his breath. He stood reluctantly.

'Five minutes. Not a second more.'

Vincent walked away in the direction of the car, pulling on his jacket. Norman knelt down and whispered in Philip's ear.

'He thinks it's going to be him ending your miserable crummy existence,' he hissed, grinding the tip of the gun barrel into Philip's temple. 'That'll be my pleasure. But first I'm going to give you something to remember me by, while you're rotting in hell!'

It wasn't only Norman's language that was lurid. He put the gun down on the ground, turned Philip roughly on to his stomach, and thrust his hands up under the back of the SS jacket. Philip felt him clawing at the zip of his corset. He had been thinking up till that point that things couldn't have got any worse. He had been wrong. The hands clawing lustily at his fasteners left no room for doubt. The time-bomb of ignominy that would explode one day at his inquest was being further primed: not only was he to be found gruesomely murdered in a state of cross-dress; he was going to be buggered senseless into the bargain first.

He bucked and writhed, trying to throw Norman off. Revulsion and shame gave him strength. This was no way for a great actor to take his curtain call. It was the most premature waste of talent since the death of Kean!

'Lie still!' Norman barked, grabbing him by the hair and banging his forehead into the dirt. 'Lie still or else!'

Or else what? Philip wondered. He summoned up his last ounce of strength, twisted his body desperately and threw Norman off.

Norman yelped as he fell against the tree stump, knocking the torch to the ground. The torch rolled gently away, the beam flickering over the fresh-dug grave. Philip lifted his left hand and wiped a thick clot of dirt away from his eye.

He had lifted his hand . . . He sat staring at it for a frozen moment before he realized what had happened. The rope must have snapped. He'd done it at last, and he hadn't even known he was still trying. His hands were free.

'You've asked for it now!' muttered Norman, staggering to his feet and lurching towards him. Philip kicked out blindly.

Norman fell on top of him. Philip felt his hot sour breath on his face, smelt the sweat and the petrol-damp shirt. He thrust out his right hand and flicked on the lighter.

Norman exploded like a Roman candle. His shirt became a sheet of flame. It engulfed his torso and leapt up to his head, rimming his few lank hairs with a burning Medusan halo. He rolled away across the grass, burning. His face had assumed the mask of a scream, but no sound came from his lips.

Vincent was shouting something, his heavy step was coming crashing through the undergrowth. Norman was throwing himself from side to side, trying to put out the flames. He was a human torch, lighting up the whole of the little clearing.

Philip's fingers closed around the butt of the black-handled revolver. He felt for the safety catch with his thumb. Was up on or off? He could never remember.

Vincent burst out of the trees and ran to Norman. He began beating the flames with his jacket. Philip was halfway across the clearing before he noticed him.

Their eyes met for one fraction of a moment. Philip saw by the flickering savage light the shock, the surprise, and then the fear. Vincent snatched at the gun in his waistband.

Philip shot him from a distance of three feet. The noise was deafening, the recoil of the gun like an animal kick. Vincent fell on to his back on the ground beside Norman. A thick dark pool of blood was spreading out from a hole in his shoulder. He stared up at Philip in blank amazement.

'Not bad for a powder puff,' said Philip, and shot him again between the eyes.

He turned the gun on Norman and fired for a third time, clinically, at the bald patch illumined like a bullseye by the smouldering hair. Norman's skull disintegrated into a jelly of brains and blood.

Philip felt nauseous. He stood swaying on his aching legs, his ears ringing painfully with the violent noise of the shots, his nostrils filled with the stink of cordite and charred flesh. He tore the remnants of the hateful gag away from his face, rubbed dolefully at his tender wrists. His whole body was a patchwork of sores and bruises. He wanted to sleep for a week. He glanced at the open grave. A week was a lot less than had been planned.

He had already pushed his body to the limit. Now he had to push it that little bit further.

He did what he had to do methodically, refusing even to acknowledge his exhaustion. He put out the burning shirt with Vincent's jacket, went through Norman's trouser pockets and found his keys. The car keys were in the jacket. He put them on the ground next to both the guns. He dragged the bodies by the ankles to the edge of the grave they had dug for him and rolled them in, one on top of the other. He replaced the torch on the tree stump so that he could see what he was doing, then he picked up the spade and filled in the grave.

The earth was loose and easy to shovel in, but it took time. He was feeble, he had to pause often for breath. He stopped too in order to listen, imagining that every creak in the night was an approaching inquisitive footstep. He had no idea where he was, how far from the nearest habitation. The thick woods would have muffled the gunshots, but they had been hideously loud. The night was his ally. Even the light of the torch could not have been visible through the trees at more than fifty yards.

There were bloodstains on the earth. He covered them with the spade. The fresh mound of the grave was harder to disguise. He threw on a few stray bits of branch and bush, but it was a token effort. It would have to do.

He picked up the guns, keys, jacket, spade and torch and returned to the car. He put the spade in the boot, and swapped his black SS jacket for Vincent's. Norman's coat was on the passenger seat. He stowed the rest of his things underneath it.

He examined his face in the car mirror. He looked as ghastly as he felt. His skin was an abstract palette of make-up, dirt and dried blood. Changing clothes was all very well, but the face was the problem, though it was a moot point whether anyone who happened to glance in would feel compelled to call the police or the Chamber of

Horrors. He examined his watch and found that it was after three o'clock. He'd take his chance. He put the key in the ignition, turned on the engine and promptly reversed into a tree.

Driving had never been one of his strong points. He'd taken his test twenty-odd years ago, but he had never owned a car. He considered them more trouble than they were worth in London, and if he couldn't take a taxi he'd go by train. He fiddled with the gearbox again and gingerly inched the car back on to the path. He seemed only to have smacked the bumper. The lights were still working.

Luckily he'd been required to drive during the filming of his last job, the aga saga, and after a near disaster on the first day the director had whisked in an instructor for some emergency refresher lessons. He was meant to be playing a curate, the director had reminded him, not Mr Toad. But he'd never in his life driven anything as big as the Volvo. It felt like a tank.

Slowly, painfully, he reversed back down the path. There was nowhere to turn, he had no choice. The faint rear lights were hardly any use at all. He drove more by luck and instinct than judgement. After about a hundred yards he drove into a five-barred gate.

He only knew that it was a five-barred gate when he got out to have a look. The Volvo hadn't even been scratched. Perhaps it was a tank. He opened the gate and reversed out into a hedged country lane. He drove away in the direction in which he found himself heading.

He didn't know whether it was the way they'd come, but after about five minutes he did rattle over a cattle grid. Shortly afterwards he came to a junction, but there was no signpost. He turned left. After another couple of miles he came to a main road, where there was a signpost. The only name on it he recognized was Harlow, and he wasn't entirely sure where that was, though he had some vague grim memory of a concrete soulless theatre. Bold blue lettering announced that there was a motorway nearby. The motorway was the M11. By the time he got into London he was almost comfortable at the wheel. He took the signs marked West End. There were more cars around than he would have thought, but whenever he had to stop he would casually lean against the door and shield his face with his hand. None of the other drivers gave any indication of having noticed him. Once he even found himself waiting for the lights to change next to a police car. His real problem was tiredness. Dogged determination kept his eyes open. He had one last matter to attend to.

It was after half past four when he drove into the mews at the back of the club. He'd have been there a little sooner had he not got lost in the unfamiliar one-way system. As he got out of the car he noticed that the office light was still on. He scurried quickly out of sight as he saw a voluminous outline take shape behind the curtain.

He let himself in through the garage using Norman's key. The stair and landing lights were on. The glass office door was slightly ajar.

'You took your time!' said Doris drily as Philip walked in.

'Better late than never,' he answered.

Doris was sitting in the chair behind the desk. Philip pointed Vincent's gun at his chest.

'The diary, please.'

Doris had gone very pale. His skin, scrubbed clean of make-up, was white already, but not a fleck of colour remained. The eyes flared for a moment with horror, then went blank.

'It's in the safe,' Doris said quietly.

'Open it.'

Doris's huge bulk seemed, perversely, almost to glide across the room. He seemed to be in a trance. The false safe door was open, as Philip had left it. Doris knelt down and reached for the inner door. He stared at the combination lock.

'Twelve-eleven-forty-six,' said Philip.

'I don't suppose you'd be interested in a deal?'

'No.'

Doris extended his arm into the safe. There was a pause. Then he spun round clumsily.

Philip shot him twice in the chest. The gun gave two tiny pops; the silencer swallowed the noise. Doris shuddered once, and never moved again. One of the bullets must have penetrated his heart.

Philip stepped over his body, and over the gun which had fallen from his hand. It was another revolver, like the Smith & Wesson. He had known Doris kept a gun in the safe, he'd heard him offer it to Vincent. He had known too that he would go for it. It didn't make any difference. He would have shot him anyway.

He picked up the revolver and added it to his collection. He was already feeling blase about guns. A few hours ago he'd never even fired one; now he was leaving a trail of destruction rarely seen outside of films by Sam Peckinpah. He must have been a natural.

The big red diary was sitting at the back of the safe, underneath the cash-box. He took them both. Doris had no need of the money any more. He also took Seymour's IOUs from the desk drawer.

He left Bosie Butterflys for the last time, laden with booty. By the time he eventually reached home dawn had broken. It had been a rough night.

212

15

Philip was asleep on the sofa when the door buzzer sounded. He rose reluctantly to press the release button. He unlocked the front door and walked stiffly to his armchair. He lit a cigarette.

Nigel Loseby appeared in the doorway, squinting. The heavy curtains were drawn, the only light was that spilling through the open door behind him.

'Philip?'

'Here. Come in.'

Nigel closed the door and pitched the room into near darkness.

'I can hardly see.'

'The tall lamp by the sofa. Turn it on.'

Nigel fumbled for the switch. When his narrowed eyes had adjusted again to the brightness they widened and filled with surprise.

'Good God, Philip! What happened to you?'

'I fell down the stairs. Have a seat.'

Nigel sat on the edge of the sofa. His manner was as it had been all along, nervous and uncertain. Clumsily he took out a packet of cigarettes.

'There's a lighter on the table,' said Philip. 'Next to the ashtray.'

Nigel lit his cigarette with Vincent Dorigo's lighter. He glanced at the butts in the ashtray.

'I didn't think you smoked.'

'I didn't.'

He'd taken his first cigarette yesterday morning, without thinking. He had finally made it home at about 7.30 a.m., having collected all his things from Conchita's flat and scrubbed out all traces of Marlene. After sprucing himself up he had put on Frank Walsingham's suit and a pair of dark glasses and left, laden with luggage, for Highbury, changing taxis three times along the way to muddy the trail. He had abandoned the Volvo in Marylebone. He was so dog tired by the time he reached home he could hardly keep his eyes open. It was then, on autopilot, that he had taken a cigarette from the gold packet sitting on the hall table.

He'd been in bed the rest of the day, apart from a brief interlude when he had visited the library. He had slept much of the night, too. It was now Sunday morning. There were only a couple of cigarettes left in the packet.

'Old habits die hard,' he murmured, half to Nigel, half to himself. 'Man cannot live by fresh air and exercise alone.'

Exercise would be a struggle at the moment; he still throbbed all over. Fresh air had been banished, with the light. He sat in a nicotine fug of his own making, enjoying the vapours, stewing in his juices. It felt good to be alive.

Nigel cleared his throat awkwardly.

'You said you had . . . something for me.'

'On the table. Brown envelope.'

He would enjoy being alive more when his body had recovered. The bruises and the soreness would go in a few days. The inner scars were another matter. He sucked on his cigarette deeply. It was balm for the nerves.

'Oh my God . . .' murmured Nigel breathlessly.

The brown envelope had fallen to the floor. He held in his hands his father's red book. His hands were clearly shaking as he opened it and began to read.

Philip watched him dispassionately. He had gone through a lot to get Seymour's diary. He had endured more

214

and acted with greater ruthlessness than at any time in his mazy dark career. To the world at large he was a distinguished and refined middle-aged Shakespearian actor; a bit of a ladies' man to some; just another thespian powder puff to others. But there was another side that the world could not have even begun to guess at. A shadow Philip, a secret sharer, supreme amoralist, criminal, killer.

'This is incredible,' said Nigel, putting down the book. 'How –?'

'Don't ask. Just take it, and go, and make sure no one else sees it.'

'Don't worry about that. I've already destroyed the others. This'll go the same way. Are you sure it's all here?'

'Why do you ask?'

'Some pages seem to have been torn out.'

'Seymour must have done that. It's all there.'

'Thank God.'

Nigel retrieved the envelope and slipped the book back inside. He hadn't stopped shaking; now it must have been with relief. He took a long time putting out his cigarette. He seemed to be collecting his thoughts.

'You saw the news yesterday, I suppose?' he said at last.

'I heard the radio. Why?'

'Well. Hm.' Nigel coughed. 'Extraordinary coincidence, but, that club, where Dad died, it burnt down. Did you know?'

Philip shrugged. Of course he knew. It had been he who had started the fire. Those petrol-stained sheets had gone up a treat. If he had left any careless stray fingerprints behind it was nothing to worry about now. Pyromania was another first for him; something else to add to his list of dubious accomplishments.

'You know they found the body of the owner, too?'

'Yes? I wasn't really paying attention.'

'Body was terribly charred, of course, but he'd been shot.'

'Ah yes, something about an open safe, wasn't there? Robbery the motive, I presume.'

'I suppose so. The other partner's disappeared, the police are looking for him. Still, it is an amazing coincidence, don't you think?'

'Why?'

'I had a call. From one of the Sunday papers. The editor said this person – the one who died – had approached him, claimed he had something to sell. Dad's diary.'

'And what did you say?'

'I said – what diary? I don't know anything about a diary.'

'And what did he say?'

'He supposed it was a con, a scam of some kind. I said I'd never met this person, I knew nothing about him. My father never kept a diary.'

Nigel Loseby picked up the thick brown envelope. He tucked it very deliberately under his arm.

'Thank you, Philip. I'll never be able to thank you enough.'

'Oh you will, Nigel, you will. Remember our deal?'

'Of course. I never renege on my promises.'

'Unique for a politician.'

Nigel laughed. He sounded quite relaxed. His old confidence was returning.

'No need to be cynical, Philip. We're not all two-faced. I'll see what I can do, put a word in the right ear. It might take a little time.'

'The state the government's in at the moment, I'm not sure you've got much time. I expect to be on the next list.'

'That may not be possible.'

'If Richard Jones's name is on it, and mine isn't, you'll be sorry.'

'Why, Philip, you're sounding petulant!'

The amused tone in Nigel's voice was put on. The tight smile expressed his irritation. He was playing the busy VIP

216

now, he had a full day's schedule, the country still needed governing even at weekends. He looked at his watch.

That little careless glance made Philip's blood boil. His battered tortured body screamed its protest from every pore. He hadn't come within a whisker of violation and extinction to be fobbed off by this oleaginous little prat.

'There are some very interesting passages in that diary, Nigel. Not all relating to Seymour. Like father, like son, eh?'

'What are you insinuating?'

'You know I never did quite swallow the whole story. Of course, what Seymour got up to was outrageous, and the blue-rinse Party stalwarts would undoubtedly be shocked, but these things blow over in time, even your political opponents might have been sympathetic. And the public isn't stupid. Your father's dubious morals can hardly be laid at your door. It's your own you should be worried about.'

'How dare you –?'

'I wondered why that tape you played me cut off in mid-flow. At a guess I'd say there was quite a bit more, wasn't there? Rather more of a reason for you to have wanted to get your hands on the diary than you were willing to let on.'

'I don't know what –'

'Try the entry for the first week of last July. Failing that, there's a very juicy bit the previous February. I couldn't quite work out whether you were still screwing your secretary then, or had you decided to concentrate all your energies on the research assistant? Lucky for you they were both so discreet. Lucky for you too that Seymour was so persuasive. The way he tells it your wife was adamant on a divorce till he came along. That would have been messy, wouldn't it? Seymour's description of the scene is exquisite, I can picture him hamming it up to the hilt as only he could – him falling to his knees, putting on his inimitable old-grey-hairs-in-sorrow-to-the-grave act and tearfully begging her to give you one last chance. Takes real acting skill to pull off an iffy scene like that. You've a lot to thank your old dad for. Saved your marriage, and – more important – saved your career. In the current climate just a whisper of the kind of sex and sleaze you've been indulging in and you'd have been out on your ear. But I don't have to spell that out for you, do I?'

'You're doing a pretty good job.'

'Gratitude, Nigel. All I want is a little gratitude. Look at me. Look at the state I'm in. I fell down a lot of bloody stairs to get that diary, and I have no intention of letting you forget it. Do we understand one another?'

'Are you making a formal threat of blackmail?'

'No, no. Let's keep it informal. Would you excuse me a moment, please?'

The telephone was ringing. When he heard the voice at the other end he experienced his first genuine frisson of pleasure in many a long day.

'You couldn't be a darling and call back in five minutes, could you?' he said into the phone. 'I've got someone with me.'

'Blonde or brunette?' came the reply.

'If it had been either I would have had better things to do than answer the telephone.'

He replaced the receiver and lit his penultimate cigarette. He took a deep drag, stretched and slumped back in an attitude of attempted repose. Nigel Loseby was staring at him morosely.

'Well?' Philip enquired.

'I'll see you get what you want.'

'What I deserve,' Philip corrected.

'What you deserve,' repeated Nigel, with some asperity. 'I sincerely hope, Philip, you get exactly what you deserve.'

'So do I, Nigel, so do I. You'll forgive me if I don't get up to see you out? Falling down those stairs has rather taken it out of me. Look after yourself. And be careful who you go to bed with.'

He sat in the semi-darkness when Nigel had gone, smoking his cigarette thoughtfully. He didn't think he could afford to fall down any more stairs, ever again. He was getting too old for this lark, this business of forever sailing close to the wind, his flag the jolly roger. It was time to come about, to view the world with a more circumspect gaze. As one soon to be elevated in rank and style he could not afford to be seen in the company of low-life and riff-raff, categories which unfortunately included most actors of his acquaintance. He would have a position to maintain, duties and responsibilities beyond mere personal requirement. As a figurehead for the British theatre he could afford only to be perceived adorning his profession.

The phone interrupted his thoughts bang on cue. Her timing had always been immaculate.

'Are you alone now?' asked Natasha.

'You're never alone with a Strand,' he answered reflectively, putting out his cigarette.

'If you're in one of your pompous moods, Philip, I don't think I can be bothered to talk to you. Where have you been, by the way? I've been trying to get through for days, and you know I'm miles from the nearest phone.'

'Oh, I've been here and there.'

'Don't try and be too communicative now, will you?'

'Is this a social call or an official interrogation?'

'I just thought you might like to know how I am, Philip.'

'And how are you, Natasha?'

'About six months pregnant with your child, since you ask.'

'Had any cravings?'

'Only to visit severe physical injury on you.'

'That's already been taken care of. Sounds like you're missing me, then?'

'Like a fly misses a dungheap.'

'Did you ring only to insult me?'

'No, I just thought I'd get that bit out of the way first. I understand you spoke very movingly at Seymour's funeral. I'm sorry I couldn't be there.'

'We gave him a pretty fair send-off.'

'Dear, darling Seymour. It's hard to believe he's no longer with us.'

'In a way he still is.'

'It's not like you to wax metaphysical.'

'That's not what I meant. Did you know he kept a diary?'

'Doesn't everybody?'

'I don't mean an appointments book. He made a note of everything. And you know what a gossip he was. He scribbled down every last little piece of innuendo.'

'You've seen it, have you?'

'I've got it here.'

He lifted out a box-file from underneath the pile of magazines on the table and clicked it open. It was filled with the pages he had painstakingly photocopied yesterday in the library, neatly bound together with rubber bands. On top was the gun from the safe with which Doris had intended to shoot him, and on top of that some half-dozen pages in Seymour's original ink, the ones he had torn out before returning the diary to Nigel. He lifted them out of the box-file.

'Remember the day after you'd done away with Sergei?' he asked.

'Don't put it like that. It's so indelicate.'

'I'm not sure there is a delicate way to discuss murder. Anyway, we had a bit of a row in my dressing room, if you recall. Well, it turns out Seymour was in his dressing room at the time, next door. Very poor quality sound-proofing backstage at the Riverside, apparently.'

'Are you saying he heard every word?'

'Enough to put two and two together and make about

three and three-quarters. He knew we were having an affair.'

'But we hadn't even done it then.'

'A technical detail. As he noted in his diary, the intensity of our quarrel could only possibly mean that we were lovers. It turns out the police were not the only ones who suspected us of being up to no good. Remember the party he gave at the end of the show? Apparently that was when he confirmed for sure we were an item. I'm afraid we weren't nearly as discreet as we thought.'

'Canny old Seymour! Good God, Philip, if any of this gets out it could be dangerous.'

'It won't. I've got the only copy.'

'How did you manage that?'

'That – as they say – is a long story.'

'You know, I do miss you sometimes.'

'As a fly does a dungheap?'

'A figure of speech. It's beautiful out here, the lakes, the mountains. Still, I can't wait to be back in London. With our child.'

'You're not proposing we play Happy Families, are you?'

'Of course not, you know it has to stay a secret.'

'Let's hope no one else is keeping a diary.'

'There was only one Seymour. You know, I've a sneaking suspicion you might make rather a good father.'

'Well, don't whisper it abroad; my reputation will never recover.'

'You'd make a lousy husband, though.'

'On that we are agreed.'

'You can take him to football matches when he grows up.'

'I've never taken anyone to a football match in my life and I have absolutely no intention of starting now. Besides, I thought you were convinced it was going to be a girl?'

'I'm not so sure any more. It's got a hell of a kick.'

'So have a number of women of my acquaintance.'

It was another forty minutes before he put down the phone again. They had a lot to talk about. If there was anyone he could trust in his shadow world it was Natasha. Had she been around in the last few days he didn't think he'd have got into quite the same degree of mess. He wished she could have been with him now. He felt a pang inside when at last their conversation ceased.

'Must be going soft in my old age,' he murmured, rising stiffly and carrying the box-file over to the coffee table. He'd take it down to the safe deposit box in a day or two. The photocopy was his insurance, a prompt for young Nigel in case of forgetfulness. As for the gun, it wouldn't do any harm just having it there, in case of emergency. The two which he had fired were in a waste skip at the back of King's Cross, along with various props and items of costume. He had covered his tracks thoroughly. Only one incriminating item of evidence remained.

He glanced through the six original diary pages one last time. All the author's suspicions were confided there, along with a deal of material which he had not mentioned to Natasha. The subject of Philip Fletcher had been a recurrent theme of Seymour's.

'Not very flattering about me, were you?' he murmured, scanning the lines of faded violet ink for barbed remarks. ' "If Philip were only half as good as he thinks he is he'd be better than Olivier, Gielgud and Richardson rolled into one. He acts as if he's God's gift to the English theatre. Conclusive proof that the Almighty has a sense of humour." Oh, very amusing, Seymour, dear! "Philip is a sick character in search of an ego" – that's choice, isn't it? And to think of all the kind words I wasted on your oration! How about this – "If Philip's innocent then so was Jack the Ripper"? That was the time when Richie died. You thought I'd done it, but then, you did seem to think I'd done everything. Well, sometimes I had, and sometimes I hadn't . . .'

He knelt down, flicked on Vincent Dorigo's lighter and set the corners of the sheets on fire. The flames spread quickly, devouring the violet words. He dropped the smouldering ball of paper into the ashtray.

'Goodbye, old friend. Ashes to ashtray, trust to dust . . .'

His haunches ached. Not that it made any difference: all of him still ached. He would go back to bed now; he could recuperate at his own pace. There had been a message from his agent on the answerphone, relaying a job offer from Chichester. He'd think it over in bed, but he knew that he was going to say yes. It would be a relief to tread the boards again in conventional costume and make-up. There'd be time for a holiday before rehearsals. He needed it. Perhaps he'd visit the Algarve after all. He might even see about a trip to Canada. He could afford to treat himself. There had been about £4,000 in the Bosie Butterflys cash-box.

He rose and stretched his stiff limbs. He caught a glimpse of his face in the glass of the coffee table.

'Arise . . .' he murmured with a regal intonation.

He smiled at his ghostly reflection.

'Arise, Sir Philip Fletcher . . .'